James M. Holbertmys

Renal Biopsy

Renal Biopsy

D. B. BREWER
M.D.(Path.)Lond., F.R.C.Path.

Professor of Morbid Anatomy, University of Birmingham
Honorary Consultant Pathologist, United Birmingham Hospitals
and Birmingham Regional Hospital Board

Second Edition

The Williams & Wilkins Company
Baltimore

SANS TACHE

© D. B. Brewer, 1973

First published 1964
by Edward Arnold (Publishers) Ltd.
25 Hill Street, London W1X 8LL

Second edition 1973

ISBN: 0 7131 4207 3

Printed by William Clowes & Sons, Ltd., London, Colchester and Beccles

Preface to Second Edition

The intention in preparing the second edition has been the same as that in preparing the first edition, to produce a guide to renal disease based on my personal experience.

All the clinical histories of the illustrated cases have been brought up to date. For this I am grateful to Dr. J. D. Blainey and Professor J. Hardwicke.

Chapters 2, 3 and 4 have been extensively rewritten to include recent advances. In addition the published work on the quantitative assessment of renal biopsies is discussed in the hope that it may ultimately provide a solution to some of our diagnostic difficulties.

A short technical appendix is included in response to many enquiries I received. It gives details of a method of cutting 1 μm section developed by the technical staff at the General Hospital, Birmingham.

Birmingham, 1973   D.B.B.

Acknowledgements

The high quality of the illustrations is due to the skill and care in preparing the sections for which I am particularly grateful to Mr. Allan Ayres at the General Hospital Birmingham and Mrs. B. Cox in the Department of Pathology, University of Birmingham. I am also grateful to Mr. S. Gaunt, Department of Pathology, University of Birmingham who took most of the photomicrographs and to Miss G. L. Parkinson who typed the manuscript.

Figures 5.5–5.9 are published with the permission of Professor C. L. Oakley, Editor of the Journal of Pathology and Bacteriology. I am grateful to Professor W. T. Smith, Professor of Neuropathology, University of Birmingham, for fig. 8.10.

Contents

I

The Development, Limitations and Complications
of Renal Biopsy

Renal biopsy is now an important part of the investigation of renal disease. With modern techniques it is a reasonably safe procedure and is regularly used in all centres where renal disease is studied. Its use, combined with careful clinical and functional studies, has added greatly to our knowledge of a wide range of diseases of the kidney and it provides tissue which is suitable for modern histochemical and electron microscope investigations which cannot be pursued on autopsy material.

The investigation has its limitations. The sample of tissue obtained is small, but despite the early doubts of pathologists proves adequate in a majority of cases. The procedure is not entirely without risk as will be discussed later in this chapter and often does not provide knowledge of value to the individual patient immediately concerned. Therefore it would seem best the investigation should be undertaken in circumstances where the biopsy material will be fully studied and correlated with complete clinical investigations of the patient.

History of renal biopsy

Before 1943 there were only a small number of reports of histological studies of the kidney during the life of the patient. These were based on open surgical biopsies usually done incidentally during some other surgical procedure. Thus Gwyn (1923) strongly advocated making the most of such opportunities, he said 'a kidney can always suffer the loss of a millimetre of substance: the upper surface of an enlarged liver away from the intestine might spare a sliver'. He performed biopsies of the kidney in 2 cases, one being a case of nephrotic syndrome in which the biopsy showed renal amyloidosis. The patient subsequently survived 7 years dying eventually of a spreading cellulitis. This biopsy must presumably have been performed about 1916.

Dorothy Russell (1929) in her classic monograph on Bright's disease included 8 cases in whom biopsies of the kidney had been performed during decapsulation. She later (1934) described a case in which the changes found at post-mortem examination in 1932 were compared with the early manifestations of the disease found in the kidney removed surgically in 1916, a case foreshadowing the value of renal biopsy in elucidating the natural history of renal disease.

In 1943 Castleman and Smithwick published the first systematic study using renal biopsy. Kidney tissue was taken during the course of splanchnic sympathectomy for hypertension in a series of 100 patients and the degree of vascular change was assessed. From these studies they found that the degree of vascular damage was much less than that usually seen in similar patients at autopsy. They concluded that in more than half the cases the vascular changes were insufficient to be the sole factor in producing hypertension and that in many cases the hypertension probably antedated the renal vascular lesion.

The first systematic attempt at *needle* biopsy of the kidney appears to be that of Nils Alwall. The biopsies were performed in 1944 but not reported until 1952. Biopsy was attempted in 13 patients. Sufficient kidney tissue was obtained in 10. Unfortunately 1 patient suffering from oliguria and uraemia died following biopsy and because of this Alwall abandoned the technique.

Iversen and Brun resumed the method and published their results in 1951 in a paper which stimulated the widespread adoption of the method.

The adequacy of the biopsy

Goldblatt criticised the paper of Castleman and Smithwick (1943) because he thought that the sample of kidney, $6 \times 5 \times 4$ mm, was too small to provide a true picture of the state of the renal vessels.

In a later study (1948), when their series had increased to 500 patients they answered this criticism by showing that their assessment of the renal vascular change was consistent and correlated well with clinical manifestations of the disease. In 100 patients biopsies were taken from both kidneys. In 95 per cent of these cases the vascular disease for all practical purposes was identical in the 2 biopsies. There was good correlation between the degree of vascular change and renal function as studied by phenolsulphthalein excretion and measurement of renal plasma flow. There was also fairly good correlation between the biopsy grades and the retinal vessel changes when the lowest and highest grades were considered.

The biopsies obtained by needle puncture have similarly been criticised as being too small, probably with rather more justification than open biopsies. Needle biopsies obviously vary much more in size than surgical biopsies. On some occasions no tissue is obtained. Thus Alwall in his pioneer series obtained tissue in 10 of 13 patients. Iversen and Brun using a similar technique with the patient in a sitting position obtained tissue in 42 of 62 patients in 80 attempts. They later abandoned their method and following Kark performed the biopsy in the prone position with a considerable increase in the number of successful biopsies. Thus Brun and Raaschou (1958) gave the figures for 510 attempts at biopsy. In the first 267 in the sitting position 40 per cent were successful. In the subsequent 243 in the prone position 67 per cent were successful. Kark *et al.* (1958) obtained satisfactory specimens in 80 per cent of their first 500 attempts at biopsy. In recent years the proportion of successful biopsies has improved even further. A survey by Welt in 1967 of the experience of 21 leading nephrology centres gave a success rate of 89·8 per cent above the age of 14 and 93·5 per cent below 14.

Hamburger (1958) exposes the kidney by a surgical incision and then takes a biopsy from it with a needle. This is obviously a more formidable procedure than percutaneous needle biopsy but tissue is obtained in every case and the kidney can be inspected for haemorrhage on completion of the biopsy.

Raaschou (1954) found in 82 successful biopsies that the length of the tissue varied from 1 to 27 mm (average 10 mm) and the number of glomeruli per section from 0 to 35 (average 10·5).

Berger, de Montera and Galle (1961) following the techniques of Hamburger said in a series of 100 biopsies in nephrotic syndrome that almost all the biopsies they examined contained more than 20 glomeruli.

The adequacy of the biopsy depends not only on its size but also of the nature of the disease being investigated. If the disease involves the kidney diffusely obviously it is more likely to be revealed in a small biopsy than if the disease is focally distributed. Thus Kellow *et al.* (1959) compared orthodox histological sections taken at post-mortem with tissue taken from the kidney with a biopsy needle also after death. In several different diffuse conditions the correct diagnosis was made in from 100 to 63 per cent of cases, in focal conditions the results again varied with the nature of the condition from 86 to 31 per cent.

Occasionally it is possible to arrive at a diagnosis from a single glomerulus (fig. 1.1) so that even the most unpromising material must be completely examined by the pathologist.

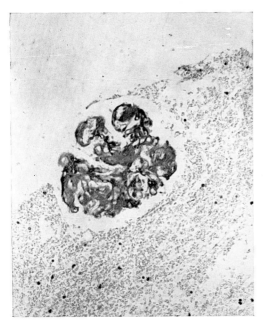

Fig. 1.1. A single glomerulus mixed with blood, the only one in the biopsy, but showing amyloidosis. PAS × 150.

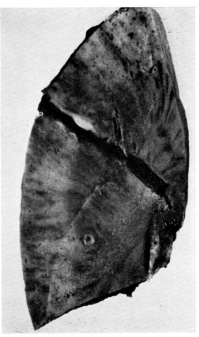

Fig. 1.2. Needle track running from cortex into medulla.

Complications of renal biopsy

It is difficult to arrive at an exact estimate of the incidence of complications following renal biopsy. Many cases go unreported and the groups of workers who have carefully recorded their experience in this respect are generally those whose care and skill make it likely that their results represent the lowest complication rates.

Bleeding is the most important common complication. It may take the form of gross haematuria, or perirenal haematoma. Blood transfusions may be required or even rarely nephrectomy.

Kark *et al.* (1958) in their first 500 biopsies found gross haematuria in 5·2 per cent of cases, perirenal haematoma in 0·6 per cent of cases. Transfusion was required in 0·4 per cent of cases, but no nephrectomy had to be performed and there were no deaths. In Brun and Raaschou's (1958) series of 510 attempts there was gross haematuria in 7·9 per cent of cases. Transfusion was required in 2·2 per cent of cases and again there were no deaths.

Experience from a wider field is recorded in the general discussion of the Ciba Symposium on Renal Biopsy (1961). The participants estimated that between them they had performed 5,120 biopsies in 15 centres. (This total includes the series of Kark *et al.* and Brun and Raaschou.) There were no deaths, but Hamburger said that he knew of 4 deaths that had occurred and had not been published. In one case in the 5,120 a kidney had had to be removed and there were 34 cases (0·6 per cent) of large perirenal haematomata.

Welt (1967, cited by Kark, 1968) recently enquired into the incidence of complications by sending a questionnaire to 21 leading nephrology centres. The total number of biopsies at all the centres was 8,081, 6,699 in patients above the age of 14 and 1,382 below the age of 14. The success rate in obtaining tissue has already been mentioned. It was 89·8 per cent of the 6,699 biopsies performed above the age of 14 and 93·5 per cent of the 1,382 below the age of 14. There were 6 fatalities (0·07 per cent).

Haematuria was the commonest complication and its incidence varied from 10 to 40 per cent. Haematuria and haematoma formation were more severe and were commoner in patients with uraemia, severe hypertension and diffuse connective tissue disorders. There were 16 haematomas and 5 nephrectomies had to be performed (0·06 per cent).

Organs other than the kidney were damaged only very infrequently. One operation had to be performed to repair a laceration of the liver. On 2 occasions splenectomy had to be performed. On 1 occasion each, the gall bladder, ureter, colon and lung were perforated. Tissue other than kidney obtained included spleen, liver and pancreas.

Serious bleeding most probably results from the needle passing through the cortico-medullary junction of the kidney and damaging the arcuate vessels (figs. 1.2 and 1.3). The arcuate artery and vein are closely adherent to one another (fig. 1.4) so that it is not surprising that occasionally arteriovenous fistulae are produced but considering the very close relationship of the artery to the vein the incidence of this complication appears to be very low. Blake *et al.* (1963) found 2 cases in a series of 62, an incidence of 3·2 per cent but Welt's enquiry revealed only 5 cases in the 8,081 biopsies, an incidence of 0·06 per cent.

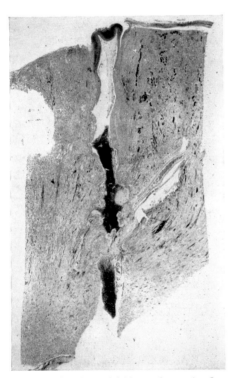

Fig. 1.3. Section of kidney shown in fig. 1.2. Needle track running close to vessels at cortico-medullary junction. HE × 4·5.

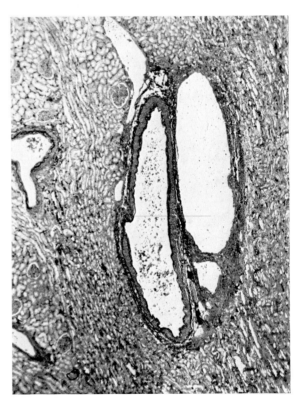

Fig. 1.4. Artery and vein at cortico-medullary junction closely adherent to one another. Elastic and van Gieson × 24.

REFERENCES

ALWALL, N. (1952). *Acta med. scand.* **143**, 430.

BERGER, J., DE MONTERA, H. and GALLE, P. (1961). *Arch. Anat. Path.* **9**, 313.

BLAKE, S., HEFFERMAN, S. and MCCANN, P. (1963). *Brit. med. J.* **1**, 1458.

BRUN, C. and RAASCHOU, F. (1958). *Arch. intern. Med.* **102**, 716.
CASTLEMAN, B. and SMITHWICK, R. H. (1943). *J. Amer. med. Assoc.* **121**, 1256.
CASTLEMAN, B. and SMITHWICK, R. H. (1948). *New Engl. J. Med.* **239**, 729.
CIBA FOUNDATION SYMPOSIUM (1961) *Discussion in Renal Biopsy*, p. 371. Churchill, London.
GWYN, N. B. (1923). *Canad. med. Ass. J.* **23**, 820.
HAMBURGER, J. (1958). *Présse méd.* **66**, 1451.
IVERSEN, P. and BRUN, C. (1951). *Amer. J. Med.* **11**, 324.
KARK, R. M. (1968). *J. Amer. med. Ass.* **205**, 220.
KARK, R. M., MUEHRCKE, R. C., POLLAK, V. E., PIRANI, C. E. and KIEFE, J. H. (1958). *Arch. intern. Med.* **101**, 439.
KELLOW, W. F., COTSONA, M. J., CHOMET, B. and ZIMMERMAN, H. J. (1959). *Arch. intern. Med.* **104**, 353.
RAASCHOU, F. (1954). *Ciba Foundation Symposium on the Kidney*, p. 15. Churchill, London.
RUSSELL, DOROTHY S. (1929). M.R.C. Spec. Rep. Series no. 142.
RUSSELL, DOROTHY S. (1934). *J. Path. Bact.* **38**, 179.

2
The Normal Kidney

In examining biopsies of kidney a detailed knowledge of the normal histological appearances is essential. It is also important to know how the appearances change, as for example, with continued post-natal development in childhood or, with incidental vascular disease in later life. A knowledge of the other abnormalities commonly found is also useful as although one is looking for deviations from an ideal normal, having discovered such changes, one then has to assess their significance. The knowledge that an appearance, although abnormal, is commonly found is essential to the establishment of the significance of such changes.

Obviously renal biopsies cannot be performed in normal people. Knowledge of the normal appearances must therefore be derived from other sources. None of them is wholly satisfactory, but none should be neglected. The major source consists of post-mortem material. Due allowance must be made for post-mortem autolysis. This affects particularly the proximal convoluted tubules but other structures probably undergo changes that are not so obvious and may only be detected by comparison of autopsy and biopsy material. Thus an observer used to seeing epithelial crescents in post-mortem specimens will be particularly struck by the different appearance of those seen in biopsy material. The cells of the crescent appear much larger and more active in biopsies. Occasional surgical specimens, removed for a variety of reasons, are of value and much can be learnt from a careful comparison of large numbers of biopsies although none of them may be strictly normal.

Renal architecture within the biopsy

One fortunately often obtains a biopsy in which the needle track runs as in fig. 1.2 so that there is successively along the length of the biopsy renal capsule, cortex, and medulla (fig. 2.1). Rarely the needle may run just below and parallel to the renal capsule (fig. 2.2) so that the biopsy will consist of subcapsular cortex and may have renal capsule along one surface (fig. 2.3). Any orientation of the biopsy track (fig. 2.4) between these two extremes may occur. In judging the effects of this it must be remembered that the renal cortex consists alternately of medullary rays running at right angles to the capsule, and made up of loops of Henle and collecting tubules and areas of cortical labyrinth containing the glomeruli, proximal and distal tubules. When the track of the biopsy needle runs obliquely into the kidney the medullary rays run obliquely across the biopsy. It is sometimes helpful to note the position of the needle track in relation to the cortical pattern as in some diseases the degree of change varies at different levels in the cortex. Thus ischaemic change is more marked in the subcapsular region and in the older patients a hyalinised subcapsular glomerulus is probably of no significance. In membranous glomerulonephritis the glomerular damage tends to be more marked in the inner cortex (Rich, 1957).

The glomerulus

This complex structure is made up of a tuft of complexly intertwined thin-walled capillaries formed from branching of the afferent arteriole and combining to form the efferent arteriole.

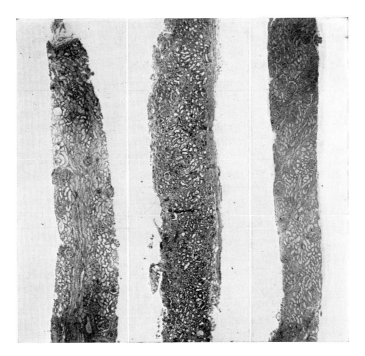

Fig. 2.1. Needle biopsy which runs at right angles to capsule. Medullary ray runs in long axis. HVG × 16.

Fig. 2.3. Needle biopsy running parallel to capsular surface with capsule along one edge. HVG × 16.

Fig. 2.4. Needle biopsy with medullary rays running obliquely across it. PAS × 24.

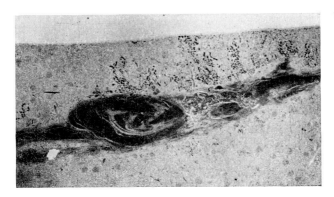

Fig. 2.2. Post-mortem specimen. Needle track filled by recent haemorrhage running almost parallel to capsular surface. HE × 8.

The capillaries rarely appear circular in cross-section in normal glomeruli even when cut transversely. Many capillaries are cut obliquely so they appear as irregularly curved, and sometimes branched, structures outlined by the glomerular basement membrane, which is also irregularly curved and infolded (fig. 2.5). The commonest condition in which the outline of the capillaries is smoother and rounder is severe congestion of the kidney although some observers (Dunn, 1934) have attached importance to this change in nephrotic syndrome.

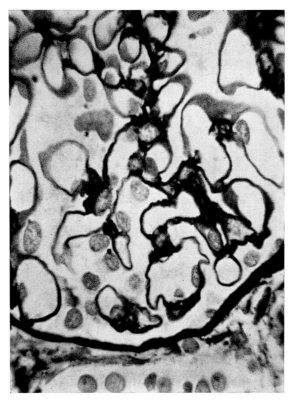

Fig. 2.5. Part of normal glomerulus showing irregular outline of capillaries. Note also the thinness of the normal glomerular basement membrane. PA silver × 900.

The capillaries arise from the afferent arteriole at the base of the tuft. Many of them appear to arise simultaneously from a little dilatation of the arteriole. This structure may in certain sections be mistaken for abnormally dilated glomerular capillaries although its true nature becomes apparent from examining serial sections (fig. 2.6). Within the tuft the capillaries are grouped in lobules. This is not generally apparent in normal tufts but often becomes obvious in disease.

The cells of the glomerulus consist of epithelial cells over the outer surface of the basement membrane of the glomerular capillaries and the inner surface of Bowman's capsule and endothelial cells and mesangial cells within the glomerular basement membrane. Epithelial cells can readily be identified by their position on the outer surface of the glomerular basement membrane. As can be demonstrated by electron microscopy the epithelial cells have a complex structure of branching cytoplasmic processes which end in numerous foot processes embedded in the

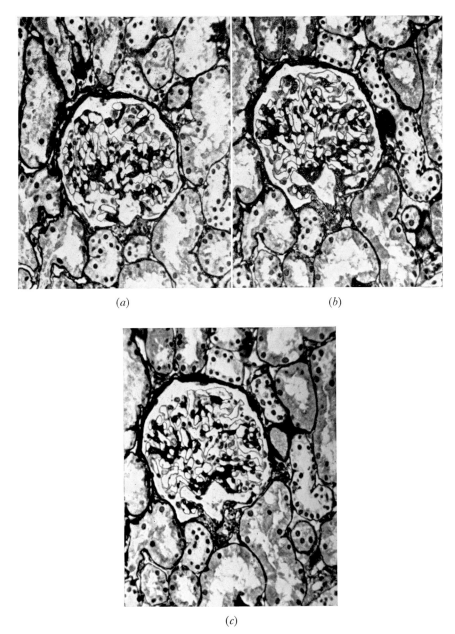

(a)   (b)

(c)

Fig. 2.6. Serial sections of a glomerulus showing afferent arteriole as it breaks up into capillaries. PA silver × 250.

basement membrane. Occasional glimpses of this arrangement can be seen with the light microscope (fig. 2.7).

It is not always possible by light microscope to identify certainly every cell within the glomerular basement membrane. Cells which have the nucleus and cytoplasm immediately adjacent to a capillary lumen are endothelial cells. This identification can be made more certain by electron

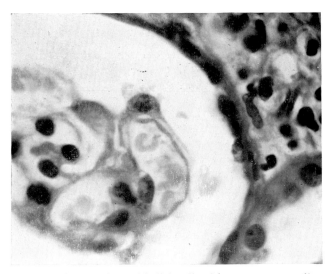

Fig. 2.7. Glomerular epithelial cell with process extending around outer surface of glomerular basement membrane. HVG × 900.

microscopy when it can be seen that these cells have a thin layer of cytoplasm lining the inner surface of the glomerular basement membrane. Other cell nuclei are seen in the centres of the lobules where small groups of capillaries meet. Most of these cells do not line capillaries and they are mesangial cells. They often proliferate in disease and become surrounded by basement-membrane-like material. They also differ from endothelial cells in that in experimental animals they readily take up injected electron-dense substances such as Thorotrast (Farquhar and Palade, 1962). Although mesangial cells differ in many respects from endothelial cells it is important to realise that they also are situated within the glomerular basement membrane. The glomerular basement membrane is pinched in at these points and does not in fact completely surround the glomerular capillary.

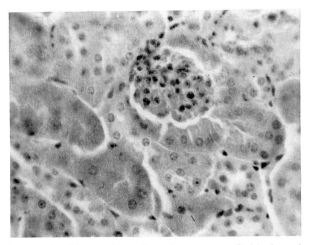

Fig. 2.8. Glomerulus of male mouse. Cubical and columnar cells lining Bowman's capsule. HE × 450.

The cells lining Bowman's capsule normally form a very flat inconspicuous layer in the human. In the male mouse these cells are cuboidal (fig. 2.8) but in the female they are squamous as in the human. It can be readily shown that this change in form in the mouse depends on the presence of male hormone (Crabtree, 1941). Similar changes have occasionally been described in renal biopsies (Finckh and Joske, 1954) without any apparent explanation.

Proximal convoluted tubules

Almost all cross-sections of tubules in the cortical labyrinth are of proximal convoluted tubules. The normal proximal convoluted tubules can readily be distinguished from distal convoluted tubules. The cells of the proximal convoluted tubules have more cytoplasm than those of the distal tubules. They also stain rather more deeply with eosin. The nuclei in the proximal convoluted tubules are more widely spaced than those of distal tubules so that fewer

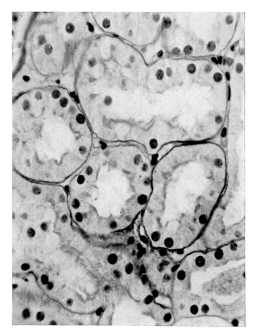

Fig. 2.9. Proximal convoluted tubules. Brush border rather irregular and incomplete. PAS × 450.

are seen in cross-sections of tubules. Other features of the cells of proximal convoluted tubules are a rather indefinite basal striation due to the orderly arrangement of the mitochondria, and a brush border on the lumenal border of the cell. This stains brightly with the PAS stain and also contains high concentration of alkaline phosphatase. One of the surprising features of biopsy material however has been the poor preservation of the border compared with animal material. The cells commonly appear to have rather a frayed edge on their lumenal border with fine loose debris apparently derived from it in the lumen of the tubule (fig. 2.9). This sort of appearance has been recognised in animal and human autopsy material by several observers over many years and has been the subject of much controversy. It is due at least in part to the formation along the brush border of spherical bodies derived from the cell cytoplasm. The bodies appear almost empty. I observed them very strikingly some years ago (Brewer, 1954) in experimental animals during the excretion of previously injected haemoglobin.

Haemoglobin fills the lumen of the proximal convoluted tubules and the spherical bodies stand out very clearly against this background (fig. 2.10). Electron microscopy of similar material in the mouse shows them to be derived from cell cytoplasm and to push through the brush border (fig. 2.11).

There has been much discussion as to whether this phenomenon (sometimes referred to as 'granuloid') is physiological or not. Bell (1950) categorically states that 'It is rather well established however, that granuloid is an artefact'. This view has recently been supported by Longley and Burstone (1963).

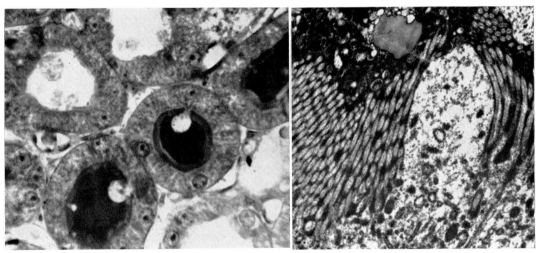

Fig. 2.10. Rat kidney after haemoglobin injection. Spherical bodies present in empty lumen of tubules and projecting into lumens filled by haemoglobin. Trichrome × 620.

Fig. 2.11. Electron micrograph of mouse kidney after haemoglobin injection Bleb of cytoplasm projecting through brush border into lumen filled with haemoglobin which appears black.

The characteristic features of the proximal convoluted tubules are often not present in diseased kidneys. This is particularly so when tubules have regenerated after previous damage. In these circumstances it may not be possible certainly to identify tubules. They can sometimes only be suspected to be proximal convoluted tubules from their number and position (fig. 2.12). In such regenerating tubules mitotic figures may be found. Multi-nucleated tubular cells are of no significance in this respect (fig. 2.13) as they are relatively common being found in 15 per cent of individuals over the age of 40 (Harman and Hogan, 1949).

The size of the lumen of the proximal convoluted tubules varies considerably. The significance of this variation has been interpreted in different ways. Rhodin (1962) until recently believed that normally there was no significant lumen, that the brush borders of adjacent cells were closely applied to one another and the glomerular filtrate percolated down the tubule between the microvilli. Now having adopted Pease's (1955) technique of fixation he agrees that there is normally a lumen. Steinhausen *et al.* (1963) demonstrated that this is so by examining the kidney by incident light microscopy in living animals. During antidiuresis for example the convoluted tubules in rats of 300 g measured 22·8 μm $\pm$ 0·7 μm in diameter. Such normal

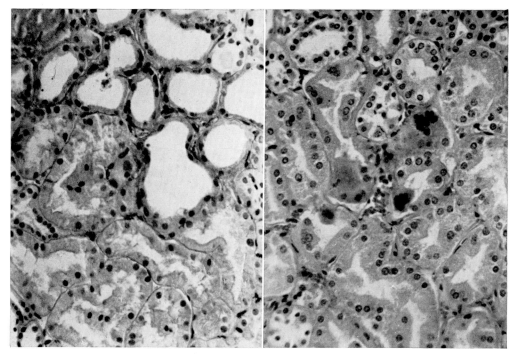

Fig. 2.12. Regenerated proximal convoluted tubules with large lumens and flat epithelium. Most of the other tubules are normal proximal convoluted tubules. PAS × 250.

Fig. 2.13. Multinucleated tubular epithelial cells. HE × 250.

tubules collapse during fixation and in sections the tubular lumens appeared much smaller. The tubules became dilated during diuresis produced by infusions of Tyrode's or mannitol solutions and did not collapse during histological processing as in the normal so that the degree of dilatation was much exaggerated.

The loop of Henle

This hair-pin-shaped loop consists of three parts. The first part is the straight portion of the proximal convoluted tubules. These tubules can be readily recognised in the medullary rays as they are lined by cells that by light microscopy appear similar to those in the convoluted portion. Electron microscopy shows them to be similar cells though rather simpler in structure. Quite suddenly in the descending limb of the loop the tubule changes in character, its lumen becomes narrower and its lining cells very flat, so flat indeed that they might be mistaken for endothelium and the tubule for a capillary (fig. 2.14). The extent of this thin portion of the loop varies but it changes again abruptly to the thick portion of the ascending limb lined by cells similar to those lining the distal convoluted tubules.

Distal convoluted tubules

The ascending limb of the loop of Henle returns to the glomerulus from which it arises and the distal convoluted tubules are adherent to the vascular pole of the glomerulus. The distal tubules are readily recognised from normal proximal convoluted tubules as they are lined by

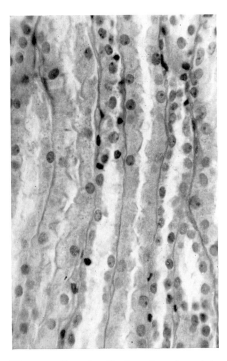

Fig. 2.14. Longitudinal section of medullary ray. Of the 4 tubules in the centre 2 are
straight portions of the proximal convoluted tubules. The other 2 lined by flattened
cells are thin loops of Henle. PAS × 450.

smaller cells with paler cytoplasm. There are more nuclei present in the cross sections of distal
tubules than proximal tubules. The distal tubules also have no brush border.

At the point of attachment of the distal tubule to the vascular pole of the glomerulus the arrangement of the tubular cells alters. They become more closely grouped on the side of the
tubule adjacent to this attachment so that the nuclei are more crowded than normal. This area
is referred to as the macula densa (fig. 2.15). The individual cells forming the macula densa
show no differences from the other cells of the distal convoluted tubule by light microscopy or
according to Rhodin (1962) by electron microscopy. However Oberling and Hatt (1960) claim
that they can be distinguished from other cells of the distal tubules by dispersion of their
mitochondria throughout their cytoplasm and by the arrangement of their basement
membrane.

The distal tubule is connected to the collecting tubule by the cortical collecting tubule (fig.
2.16). This region is of interest as it contains what Oliver (1944–45) has called 'the lost tribe of
kidney cells', the intercalated cells. These are small darkly staining cells containing meta-
chromatic granules. Their function is not known but they show a striking increase in experi-
mentally induced potassium deficiency in the rat (Oliver et al., 1957).

The large collecting ducts are lined by cubical or columnar cells with sharply defined cell
borders and clear cytoplasm. They are often not present in biopsy material. Although no
pathological changes have been described in them in man they should be examined because of
the changes described in them in potassium deficiency in the rat.

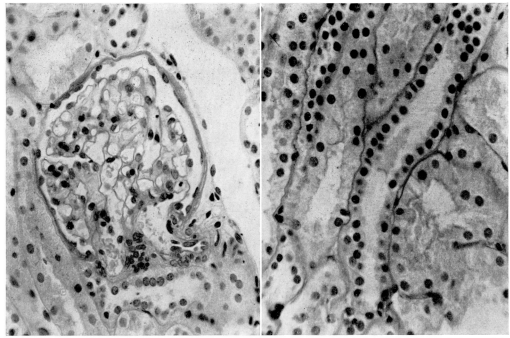

Fig. 2.15. Glomerulus with afferent and efferent arterioles. Distal convoluted tubule below with nuclei crowded to form macula densa. PAS × 370.

Fig. 2.16. Cortical collecting tubule in medullary ray. It has a large lumen and is lined by cubical cells with round nuclei. PAS × 450.

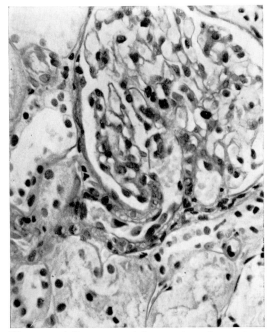

Fig. 2.17. Afferent arteriole entering glomerulus. PAS × 450.

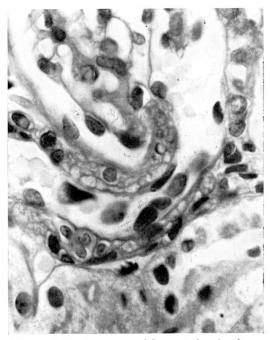

Fig. 2.18. Higher power of fig. 2.17 showing large clear cells in arteriolar media. PAS × 900.

Arteries and veins

The intrarenal arteries are muscular arteries with a single internal elastic lamina. Normally the intima is so thin to be hardly detectable.

A striking change occurs in the media of the afferent arteriole as it approaches the glomerulus. The normal spindle-shaped smooth muscle cells become replaced by cells of a more epithelial character with round nuclei and cytoplasmic granules (figs. 2.17 and 2.18). Changes in the number of these cells and their granularity have been described in experimental hypertension and in patients with hypertension so that it is probable that the cells secrete renin. The name juxtaglomerular cells or juxtaglomerular apparatus has been given to these cells but there is some confusion about the use of the term. Thus Hartroft and Newmark (1961) confine the use of the term juxtaglomerular cells to cells within the arteriolar media. Oberling and Hatt (1960) however in an interesting paper tracing the confused and controversial development of ideas regarding the structures in this area include in the juxtaglomerular apparatus the afferent arteriole, the macula densa of the distal convoluted tubules and the rather indefinite group of cells between these two structures, the polkissen of Zimmermann. Latta influenced by Oberling (Latta and Maunsbach, 1962) has accepted this definition and recently extended it (Barajas and Latta, 1962) to include the efferent arteriole on the basis of changes produced by adrenalectomy in the rat.

The assessment of renal biopsies

In most centres renal biopsies are reported in descriptive terms but commonly some attempt at a quantitative assessment of the changes present is made by use of such adjectives as slight, moderate, or severe. In recent years there have been considerable developments in statistically valid methods of making quantitative estimates of a wide variety of changes found in a variety of tissues. Such methods could with advantage be adapted to the assessment of renal biopsies, provided due consideration is given to the problem of sampling.

Good descriptions of simpler semi-quantitative methods of assessment have been published. That by Pirani and Salinas-Madrigal (1968) is very helpful in that in addition to giving guidance as to the semi-quantitative assessment of the changes found it also lists all the structures that should be examined and gives some indication of the changes to be expected in various diseases.

A method of rather more precise quantitative assessment was described by Risdon et al. (1968) in a study in which they made an assessment of glomerular change by a method of grading from 1 to 5 and assessed tubular damage by the number of fields in 10 consecutive ones that showed unequivocal tubular atrophy. They found a highly significant correlation between the extent of the tubular damage and creatinine clearance, plasma creatinine and the ability to concentrate and to acidify the urine. This rather surprising result is confirmed by Schainuck et al. (1970) in a paper in which they describe the relation between semi-quantitative assessments of histological changes, obtained by a method they describe (Striker et al., 1970) and a variety of measurements of renal function. They found good correlation between reductions in G.F.R., effective renal plasma flow, concentrating ability or ammonium excretion and the severity of tubular and interstitial changes.

Although such semi-quantitative methods are clearly capable of yielding valuable results and are closely reproducible within the group who have developed them the next important development should be the devising of more strictly quantitative methods depending on precise counting and measuring.

It is possible with a quite small amount of work to arrive at an estimate of the total number of glomeruli in a kidney (Elias and Hennig, 1967) but this requires the whole kidney so that it is impossible to do on a biopsy. This is also true of the assessment of a number of other parameters in which, from counts or measurements made on sections an estimate is made of the density of the structures under investigation per unit volume. This sample estimate can then be converted into absolute terms if the size of the kidneys is known. For example, the percentage volume of the renal cortex consisting of normal proximal convoluted tubules can readily be determined by point-counting sections, but to express the percentage in absolute terms the total volume of the renal cortex must be known.

A number of papers have been published describing attempts to arrive at some estimate of glomerular size. This is difficult problem as the spherical glomeruli are represented in sections as circles which will vary in size from the largest which is that through the centre of the sphere through a range of sizes which gets smaller the further the plane of the section is from the centre of the sphere. The diameters of the spheres, i.e. the glomeruli of which the circles are sections, will also vary about a mean. It is therefore quite a complicated undertaking arriving at an estimate of the mean glomerular size from measurements of the circles in sections. However there are several methods described of calculating the mean glomerular size from measurements made on section (Elias and Hennig, 1967).

Other simpler methods of forming some estimate of glomerular size consist of measuring the projected areas in a camera lucida drawing with a planimeter (Iidaka et al., 1968) or measuring two diameters at right angles and calculating the areas assuming the section of the glomerulus is an ellipse (Bauer and Rosenberg, 1960, Verger et al., 1966).

Counting the number of nuclei present in sections of glomeruli would seem to be a worthwhile and relatively simple procedure but from the few published results it is clearly not as simple as would first appear. Sorensen (1967) has claimed to show that variations on thickness of sections of 5, 7 and 9 μm have no effect on the total number of nuclei present. However his results for the total number of nuclei in 5 μm sections 163, 212, and 185 are considerably higher than the mean of 125·3 per glomerulus given by Iidaka et al. (1968) apparently based on 3 μm section. There is an even greater discrepancy with the results of Wehner and Anders (1969) who found a mean of only 30 cells in the glomeruli in 1 μm sections. Clearly in attempting such nuclear counts great care must be taken to standardise the techniques used.

Although the precise quantitative assessment of glomerular changes in disease may be difficult and time consuming that it can be of value is indicated by the results of two recent investigations into the glomerular changes in diabetic glomerulosclerosis. Kawano et al. (1969) using a planimetric method found that in normals the mean mesangial areas was 6·76 per cent of the total glomerular area and that it increased to 17·25 per cent in diffuse diabetic glomerulosclerosis and to 23·73 per cent in nodular diabetic glomerulosclerosis. Wehner (1968) and Wehner and Anders (1969) using a point-counting method found that in normals the mean mesangial area increased with age from 6·2 to 10·4 per cent of the total glomerular area with a mean of 8·5 per cent at the age of 42 and that in diffuse diabetic sclerosis it rose to 12·7 per cent and in nodular diabetic glomerulosclerosis to 20·7 per cent.

The methods described by Weibel (1969) in morphometric studies of the lung can readily be applied to electron micrographs of the kidney and by simple modifications to 1 μm sections examined by light microscopy.

A method of preparing 1 μm sections for light microscopy is described in the appendix.

REFERENCES

BARAJAS, L. and LATTA, H. (1963). *Lab. Invest.* **12**, 1046.
BAUER, W. C. and ROSENBERG, BARBARA F. (1960). *Amer. J. Path.* **37**, 695.

BELL, E. T. (1950). *Renal Diseases* (2nd ed.) Henry Kimpton, London. p. 20.

BREWER, D. B. (1954). *Quart. J. micr. Sci.* **95**, 23.

CRABTREE, CHARLOTTE E. (1941). *Endocrinology* **29**, 197.

DUNN, J. S. (1934). *J. Path. Bact.* **39**, 1.

ELIAS, H. and HENNIG, A. (1967). *Quantitative Methods in Morphology.* Ed. WEIBEL, E. R. and ELIAS, H. Springer-Verlag, Berlin. p. 130.

FARQUHAR, MARILYN G. and PALADE, G. E. (1962). *J. Cell. Biol.* **13**, 55.

FINCKH, E. S. and JOSKE, R. A. (1954). *J. Path. Bact.* **68**, 646.

HARMAN, J. W. and HOGAN, J. M. (1949). *Arch. Path.* **47**, 29.

HARTROFT, PHYLLIS M. and NEWMARK, J. H. (1961). *Anat. Rec.* **139**, 185.

IIDAKA, K., MCCOY, J. and KIMMELSTIEL, P. (1968). *Lab. Invest.* **19**, 573.

KAWANO, K., ARAKAWA, M., MCCOY, J., PORCH, J. and KIMMELSTIEL, P. (1969). *Lab. Invest.* **21**, 269.

LATTA, H. and MAUNSBACH, A. B. (1962). *J. ultrastruct. Res.* **6**, 547.

LONGLEY, J. B. and BURSTONE, M. S. (1963). *Amer. J. Path.* **42**, 643.

OBERLING, CH. and HATT, P. Y. (1960). *Ann. Anat. path.* **5**, 441.

OLIVER, J. (1944–45). *Harvey Lect.* **40**, 102.

OLIVER, J., MACDOWELL, MURIEL, WELT, L.C., HOLLIDAY, M. A., HOLLANDER, W., WINTERS, R. W., WILLIAMS, T. F. and SEGAR, W. E. (1957). *J. exp. Med.* **106**, 563.

PEASE, D. C. (1955). *Anat. Rec.* **121**, 701.

PIRANI, C. L. and SALINAS-MADRIGAL, L. (1968). *Path. Ann.* **3**, 249.

RHODIN, J. A. G. (1962). *Renal Diseases.* Ed. BLACK, D. A. K. Blackwell, Oxford. p. 128.

RICH, A. R. (1957). *Bull. Johns Hopk. Hosp.* **100**, 173.

RISDON, R. A., SLOPER, J. C. and DE WARDENER, H. E. (1968). *Lancet* **ii**, 363.

SCHAINUCK, L. I., STRIKER, G. E., CUTLER, R. E. and BENDITT, E. P. (1970). *Hum. Path.* **1**, 631.

SORENSEN, A. W. S. (1967). *Acta path. microbiol. scand.* **69**, 71.

STEINHAUSEN, M., IRAVANI, I., SCHUBERT, G. E. and TAUGNER, R. (1963). *Virchows Arch. path. Anat.* **336**, 503.

STRIKER, G. E., SCHAINUCK, L. I., CUTLER, R. E. and BENDITT, E. P. (1970). *Hum. Path.* **1**, 615.

VERGER, D., LELLOUCH, J. and RICHET, G. (1966). *J. Urol. Nephrol.* **72**, 318.

WEHNER, H. (1968). *Virchows Arch. Abt. A. path. Anat.* **344**, 286.

WEHNER, H. and ANDERS, E. (1969). *Ver. dtsch. Ges. Path.* **53**, 380.

WEIBEL, E. R. (1969). *Int. Rev. Cytol.* **26**, 235.

3
The Nephrotic Syndrome

With recent developments in our knowledge of the mechanisms and natural history of the nephrotic syndrome it has lost some of its mystique. The sterile exercise of hair-splitting definition of the syndrome seems now to have lost its fascination. It is now generally accepted that the essential factor in causing the syndrome is heavy proteinuria. The lowered serum albumin and severe oedema are consequences of this. They are not, however, the inevitable results of heavy proteinuria. The serum albumin falls when the urinary protein loss exceeds the capacity for protein synthesis. This is shown by the fact that it is possible in the face of very large daily losses of protein in the urine, of 15–25 g, for the serum albumin to return to levels of 3·5–4·0 g/100 ml if a very high protein diet is given (Squire *et al.*, 1962).

Nephrotic syndrome may result from any renal lesions which causes a sufficient loss of protein in the urine. The course of the disease depends on the nature of the underlying lesion as as also does the presence of hypertension or renal failure or their later development. The clinical diagnosis of the underlying kidney disease may only be possible after very prolonged observation. Renal biopsy can be of greatest assistance in rapidly making an exact diagnosis.

The Causes of nephrotic syndrome

Kark *et al.* (1958) listed 35 causes of nephrotic syndrome. Many of these must be extremely rare causes. A better idea of the main causes may be obtained from Table 3.1 which is derived

TABLE 3.1

Causes of Nephrotic Syndrome (per cent)

	Berger *et al.*	Kark *et al.*	Combined series	Spencer
Amyloidosis	6	4	10	8
Disseminated lupus erythematosus	6	19	5	4
Renal vein thrombosis	1	4	5	1
'Minimal change' glomerulonephritis	25	12	19	not included
Glomerulonephritis	48	46	47	58
Advanced lesions (not interpretable)	14	—	—	—
Diabetes mellitus	nil	14	4	23
Miscellaneous	—	1	10	6

from Lawrence *et al.* (1963) with the addition of the series reported by Berger *et al.* (1961). These series are not strictly comparable as the diagnostic criteria used are not identical and probably some selection has been exercised in collecting the cases. Such factors account for the high incidence of disseminated lupus erythematosus in the series of Kark *et al.* (1958) and the absence of diabetes mellitus from the cases of Berger *et al.* (1961).

Amyloid was the cause in 4–10 per cent of the cases and renal vein thrombosis in 1–5 per cent.

The largest group of cases by far were due to glomerulonephritis. If 'minimal change' glomerulonephritis is included amongst this group glomerulonephritis accounted for 58–73 per cent of the cases.

More detailed figures of the incidence of various forms of glomerulonephritis causing nephrotic syndrome were obtained in the recent Medical Research Council trial of steroids in nephrotic syndrome (Black *et al.*, 1970). The trial included patients over the age of 15 years who showed no clinical or pathological evidence of an underlying cause other than glomerulonephritis. Table 3.2 gives the various diagnoses in the 156 cases in which a diagnosis could be made on the biopsy material available.

TABLE 3.2

	Number	Per cent
'Minimal change' glomerulonephritis	38	24
Membranous nephropathy	25	16
Proliferative glomerulonephritis	87	56
Renal amyloidosis	6	4
Total	156	

It is interesting that even in this series in which on clinical grounds such cases should have been excluded there was still an incidence of 4 per cent due to renal amyloidosis.

'Minimal change' glomerulonephritis is much commoner in children. This is confirmed by the findings of Churg *et al.* (1970) in an international study of kidney disease in children as shown in Table 3.3. They found an incidence of 77 per cent of 'minimal change' glomerulonephritis and only 2 cases of membranous nephropathy out of a total of 127 cases.

TABLE 3.3

	Total	Per cent
'Minimal change' glomerulonephritis	98	77·0
Focal sclerotic lesions	12	9·5
Proliferative glomerulonephritis	14	11·0
Membranous nephropathy	2	1·7
Chronic glomerulonephritis	1	0·8
Total	127	

A somewhat surprising finding in the M.R.C. series was the marked differences in sex distribution in the various categories. In the 'minimal change' group the number of males and females was about equal (17 males, 14 females), but in the membranous nephropathy group there was a marked preponderance of males (16 males (84%), 3 females).

In the proliferative glomerulonephritis group up to the age of 45 there were 21 males and 20 females but above the age of 45 there were 33 males and only 1 female. It is difficult to compare the findings with published figures for proliferative glomerulonephritis as a wide variety of lesions are included under this heading. The published figures for membranous nephropathy vary considerably. Forland and Spargo (1969) found 9 males (47 per cent) and 10 females in their total of 19 cases, Pollak *et al.* (1968) 13 males (62 per cent) and 8 females in their total of 21 cases and Ehrenreich and Churg (1968) 36 males (60 per cent) and 24 females in their total of 60 cases.

Amyloidosis

Amyloidosis of the kidney is most commonly secondary. Nowadays the diseases causing it are different from those found even 20 years ago. In Bell's (1950) series of 145 cases, tuberculosis, usually pulmonary, was far and away the most important cause, accounting for 73. Because of the reduction in chronic infections other causes of amyloidosis, such as rheumatoid arthritis, have increased in importance.

Structural changes

In the kidney, as in other organs, amyloid is deposited in relation to basement membranes both of epithelial structures and of blood vessels. It is particularly prominent in the glomeruli which in advanced cases may be almost entirely replaced. It is also often marked in the veins and about the tubules in the medulla, and in the glomerular arterioles. Smaller deposits may be found about the basement membrane of the proximal tubules.

Within the glomerulus it is seen as irregularly shaped deposits of hyaline material staining brightly pink with eosin (fig. 3.1). The deposits appear to obliterate almost completely the lumen of the capillaries. The deposits seem to be limited by the glomerular basement membrane and their irregular shape follows to some extent the shape of the glomerular capillaries. The diagnosis in advanced cases is usually obvious. Occasionally it may be difficult to differentiate the change from chronic lobular glomerulonephritis or diabetic glomerular lesions. In such circumstances special stains such as methyl violet or congo red may be helpful. Congo red increases the birefringence of amyloid because the dye molecules are orientated on the fibrils of the amyloid.

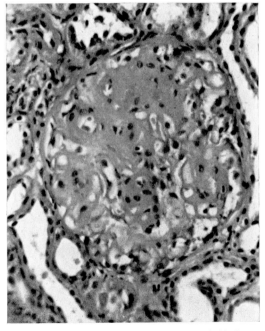

Fig. 3.1. Extensive deposits of amyloid in a glomerulus. HE × 250.

Another result of this orientation of dye molecules is the presence of anomalous colours also detectable with the polarising microscope. These are colours that can be made to change in a most striking fashion by varying the amount of compensation or more simply in an ordinary microscope fitted with Polaroid screens by rotating the slide on the stage. Similar anomalous colours are produced by staining amyloid with eosin or methyl violet (fig. 3.2).

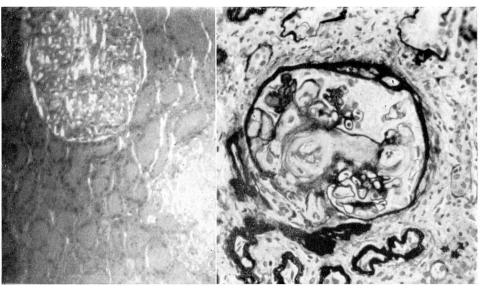

Fig. 3.2. Glomerular amyloidosis stained with eosin and photographed in polarised light.

Fig. 3.3. Glomerular amyloidosis. Basement membrane black. Amyloid only faintly stained. PA silver × 250.

The PA silver method produces a very sharp distinction between these conditions. In both diabetic nephropathy and lobular glomerulonephritis, black positively stained fibres are demonstrated at the centres of the lobules. In amyloidosis the deposits stain only very faintly and can usually be seen clearly surrounded by a black staining basement membrane (fig. 3.3).

For the demonstration of minute deposits of amyloid, fluorescence microscopy following staining with thioflavine-T (Hobbs and Morgan, 1963) is more sensitive than conventional methods. The detection of anomalous colours with the polarising microscope after staining with congo red or eosin also reveals minute deposits. In using this method however one would be assuming that all amyloid has a fibrillar structure. In any research into amyloidosis it is doubtful whether one could assume that any single method consistently demonstrated all amyloid.

The site of deposition of glomerular amyloid

There has been considerable controversy over many years regarding the exact site of deposition of amyloid in the glomerulus. These differences of opinion have continued following electron microscope investigations. Broadly there have been three views. The first is that amyloid infiltration is a consequence of a change in the substance of the glomerular basement membrane itself. This view is supported by Allen (1962) as a result of his investigations by light microscopy. Bergstrand and Bucht (1961) and Geer *et al.* (1958) support this view as a result of their investigations with the electron microscope. The difficulty obviously is to distinguish basement membrane from amyloid deposits, a difficulty which none of the supporters of this first view make any attempt to circumvent.

The two other views differ only in detail. Amyloid is thought of as something deposited on the glomerular basement membrane. Bell (1950) thought it was deposited on the inner surface, pushing the endothelial cells inwards. He said 'at no time is amyloid found external to a demonstrable basement membrane'. Undoubtedly most of the amyloid is deposited inside the capillary basement membrane but small amounts are deposited on its external surface. This has been shown most convincingly by Movat (1960) with the electron microscope using silver staining to demonstrate the glomerular basement membrane running through the deposits. It can also be seen quite strikingly in sections stained by the PA silver method in which the basement membrane stains black and the amyloid only very faintly (fig. 3.4).

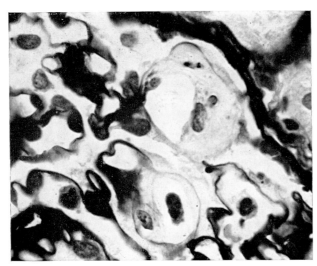

Fig. 3.4. Small portion of a glomerular tuft. Glomerular basement membrane, black. In affected capillaries basement membrane thinner and more faintly stained. Amyloid deposits on both inner and outer surfaces. PA silver × 900.

Clinical manifestations

The most important result of renal amyloidosis is proteinuria which if sufficiently severe reduces the serum albumin and causes nephrotic syndrome.

It seems probable however that the disease may be present for a considerable time before becoming clinically manifest and also the patient may survive a considerable time after the diagnosis has been made. Thus the patient of Gwyn's referred to in the first chapter survived seven years.

An interesting clinical manifestation recently reported is pituitrin-resistant diabetes insipidus (Carone and Epstein, 1960). This was in a case of renal amyloidosis in which there was relatively slight involvement of the glomeruli but cuffs of amyloid surrounded the collecting tubules in the medulla. Unfortunately it is only infrequently that the medullary collecting tubules are included in a biopsy.

Obviously renal biopsy could be of greatest help in settling the question of whether amyloid deposits regress when their cause is removed. There are occasional reports claiming that this happens (e.g. Rosenblatt, 1936) but the evidence is not entirely convincing. Biopsy confirmation of this is desirable, particularly in view of Richter's (1954) work on experimental amyloidosis showing that splenic deposits were reabsorbed but those in the kidneys were not.

Renal amyloidosis and renal vein thrombosis

There is good evidence of an increased tendency to renal vein thrombosis in renal amyloidosis. Barclay *et al.* (1960) describe a series of 9 cases and list 39 previously reported cases. The effect of this thrombosis may be either to determine the onset of nephrotic syndrome or cause a rapid deterioration in the condition of the patient with uraemia and oliguria. The exact relationship of the thrombosis to the development of the nephrotic syndrome in renal amyloidosis has not been established, but it is highly probable that nephrotic syndrome can occur without thrombosis.

Renal vein thrombosis

Renal vein thrombosis is sometimes found in cases of nephrotic syndrome without renal amyloidosis. In many of these cases changes in the glomerulus indistinguishable from chronic membranous nephropathy both by light and electron microscopy are found. The exact interpretation of this association is uncertain but the view was commonly put forward that the primary event was thrombosis of the renal veins which then caused the nephrotic syndrome and the structural changes in the glomerulus. However it is quite clear that the opposite view, that is, that the primary condition is chronic membranous nephropathy and that renal vein thrombosis is a complication of this is equally tenable.

The condition is well reviewed by Rosenmann *et al.* (1968). They describe a total of 15 cases, 11 typical and 4 with atypical features. The common histological findings were enlarged glomerular tufts, dilated glomerular capillary lumens, mild to moderate thickening of the glomerular basement membrane, intraglomerular leukocyte stasis, tubular atrophy and interstitial oedema and fibrosis. None of these features is diagnostic but they stress the importance of the findings of tubular atrophy, interstitial oedema and fibrosis which is more severe than would be expected from the degree of glomerular damage. They found such changes in 5 of their 15 patients. They were able to form some impression of the mode of progression of the changes by examining specimens obtained within 4 months of onset of the disease and specimens obtained 4 to 13 months after onset. In 6 instances they were able to examine 2 biopsies taken at an interval in the same patient. On this basis they suggest that the early changes consist of mild glomerular basement membrane thickening, glomerular leukocyte stasis and interstitial oedema and that with the passage of time interstitial fibrosis and tubular atrophy predominate. Of the 4 cases I have examined 2 have shown a similar progression of the changes.

Case 1. This was case 1 of Blainey *et al.* (1954). The sections of kidney were also examined and described by Pollak *et al.* (1956). He was a man of 70 with gross generalised oedema, proteinuria 6–10 g daily, and serum albumin 1·9 g per 100 ml. Whilst in hospital he developed signs and symptoms of pulmonary infarction and then developed renal failure. Post-mortem examination showed an infarct in the right lower lobe of the lung, an embolism in the left main pulmonary artery, and well organised thrombus in the external, internal and common iliac veins and the inferior vena cava up to and involving the renal veins. Both renal veins appeared totally occluded. The kidneys were of normal size.

Histological appearance of the kidney. All the glomeruli show diffuse thickening of the basement membrane. Although not grossly thickened the basement membrane is unusually sharp and clear (fig. 3.5). The glomerular capillaries are not congested, but, as noted by Pollak *et al.* (1956) there are polymorphs present. Although not numerous there are quite conspicuous small collections of polymorphs in about one-third to one-quarter of the tufts. The proximal convoluted tubules show only moderate post-mortem changes (fig. 3.6) and for a man of 70 there is no significant increase in interstitial tissue.

Case 2. A woman of 27 developed proteinuria during pregnancy. Following delivery 3 months later the oedema became very severe. She also suffered several pulmonary emboli.

Post-mortem examination showed organising thrombus in both renal veins extending to within 1·5 cm of their junction with the inferior vena cava. There was thrombus throughout both ovarian veins, in the

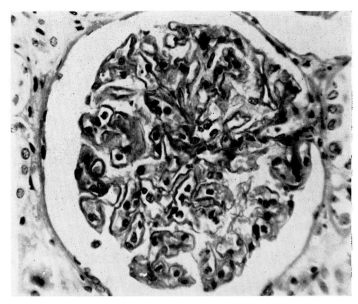

Fig. 3.5. Renal vein thrombosis. Case 1. Glomerulus showing diffuse thickening of basement membrane. PAS × 450.

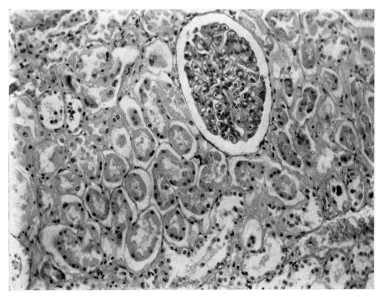

Fig. 3.6. Renal vein thrombosis. Case 1. Glomerulus and tubules. Tubules show some post-mortem change but there is no tubular atrophy or interstitial fibrosis. PAS × 150.

uterine veins on the right side of the uterus and there was thrombosis of the lower 3 cm of the inferior vena cava extending down through the right common iliac, right external iliac to the right femoral vein. Both kidneys were diffusely enlarged with pale, widened cortices.

Histologically, there is no diffuse thickening of the glomerular basement membrane but many glomeruli show small areas of adhesions with slight epithelial cell proliferation and small areas of focal

PAS positive thickening suggestive of healed focal glomerulonephritis (fig. 3.7). The proximal convoluted tubules are not obviously atrophic though minor degrees of change might be obscured by post-
mortem autolysis.

The other two cases showed at autopsy the changes described by Pollak *et al.* (1956) but they
are of great interest as biopsies taken some years earlier did not show these changes.

Case 3. Thrombosis of the right femoral vein followed the using of a breast drill pressed against the
right groin in a man of 27. The nephrotic syndrome then developed and thrombosis of the inferior
vena cava was diagnosed. He was treated with a high protein diet, anticoagulants and cortisone. He was
under treatment for 7 years and was finally admitted to hospital complaining of chest pain, nausea and
vomiting. He was uraemic and the blood pressure was 205/135 mm.

At autopsy there was marked oedema. The heart weighed 460 g and showed a fibrinous pericarditis.
In the inferior vena cava were numerous venous bands and webs extending from just above the renal

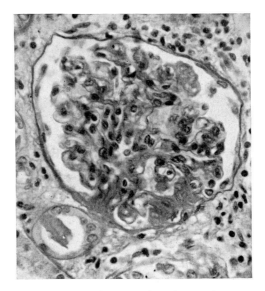

Fig. 3.7. Renal vein thrombosis. Case 2.
Glomerulus with area of irregular thickening.
PAS × 450.

veins right down into the femoral veins. There were venous bands in the right renal vein but the left
renal vein showed no evidence of previous thrombus. The kidneys were only slightly reduced in
size.

Histological findings. The biopsy taken within about a month of onset shows moderate diffuse thickening of the glomerular basement membrane (fig. 3.8). The tubules are only slightly dilated and there is no
significant interstitial fibrosis. The kidneys at post-mortem show advanced changes complicated by
severe hypertensive damage. There is severe interstitial fibrosis and complete hyalinisation of many
glomeruli (fig. 3.9). Those not completely hyalinised show marked thickening of the glomerular basement membrane (fig. 3.10).

Case 4. At the age of 46 this man sprained his ankle and sustained a small fracture. His ankle was
quite swollen but the swelling slowly subsided. About 1½ months later he noticed his eyes were swollen
in the mornings. After another month both ankles became swollen and proteinuria was discovered.
After a further 2 months a renal biopsy was performed. At this time proteinuria varied from 9·1 to 21·4 g
daily, total serum proteins 3·2 g per 100 ml, albumin 1·0 g per 100 ml, and the creatinine clearance was
59 ml per min.

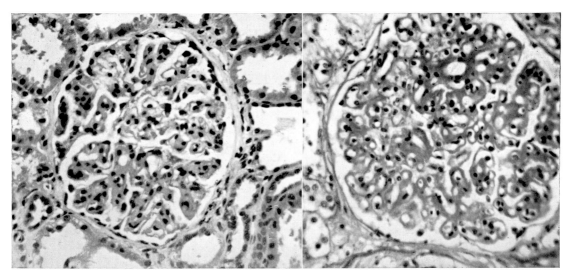

Fig. 3.8. Renal vein thrombosis. Case 3. Glomerulus in biopsy. Moderate diffuse thickening of glomerular basement membrane. No tubular atrophy or interstitial fibrosis. PAS × 250.

Fig. 3.10. Renal vein thrombosis. Case 3. Post-mortem kidney. Extensive hyalinisation of glomeruli, complete in some tufts Severe tubular atrophy and interstitial fibrosis. PAS × 100.

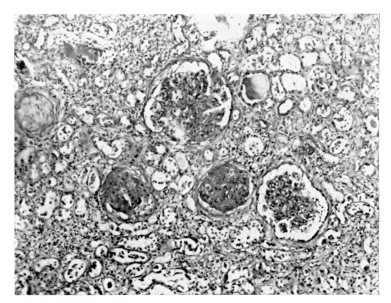

Fig. 3.9. Renal vein thrombosis. Case 3. Post-mortem kidney. Marked diffuse thickening of glomerular basement membrane. PAS × 250.

The biopsy, which contains 12 glomeruli, shows no thickening of the glomerular basement membrane. There is very slight centrilobular thickening with small areas of increased cellularity (fig. 3.11). There is one very small group of polymorphs in one glomerulus. The proximal convoluted tubules are normal and there is no increase in interstitial tissue about them. Some of the distal tubules however are slightly dilated by PAS positive casts. About these tubules there are small interstitial scars of loose fibrous tissue.

One year later a second biopsy was performed. His proteinuria was slightly less, 8–9 g daily. The total serum proteins were 3·8 g per 100 ml, serum albumin 1·43 g, and creatinine clearance 47 ml per min.

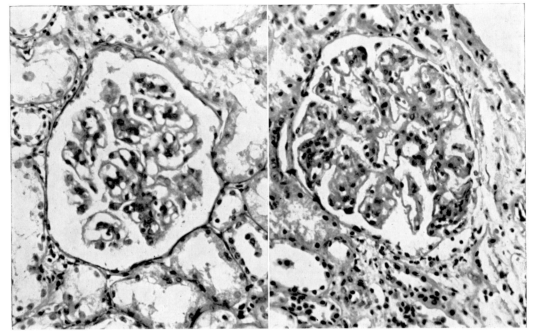

Fig. 3.11. Renal vein thrombosis. Case 4. 1st biopsy. No diffuse thickening of glomerular basement membrane. Some centrilobular thickening. No tubular atrophy or interstitial fibrosis. PAS × 250.

Fig. 3.12. Renal vein thrombosis. Case 4. Second biopsy. Slight, but definite, thickening of glomerular basement membrane. PAS × 250.

Unfortunately the second biopsy only contains four glomeruli, but they all show slight but quite definite thickening of the glomerular basement membrane (fig. 3.12). There was however no increase in interstitial fibrous tissue.

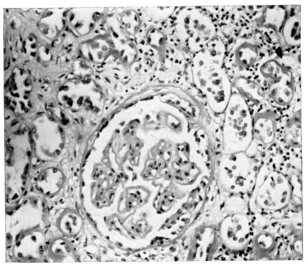

Fig. 3.13. Renal vein thrombosis. Case 4. Post-mortem kidney. Marked thickening of glomerular basement membrane, atrophy of tubules and interstitial fibrosis. PAS × 150.

After this biopsy he showed no sustained improvement. The proteinuria increased up to 18–25 g daily. The serum albumin level varied but never rose above 1·95 g per 100 ml, and the creatinine clearance fell slightly to levels of 20–30 ml per min. He died 2½ years after the onset of the disease.

Post-mortem examination showed pulmonary oedema, an old organising thrombus in the right main pulmonary artery, the kidneys each weighed 280 g. There was old partly calcified thrombus obstructing the left renal vein. The right renal vein appeared to be patent but near its orifice there was a small calcified nodule.

Histologically, the kidneys show all the glomeruli to be severely affected. All show marked thickening of the glomerular basement membrane. There are no obvious polymorphs in the glomerular capillaries. There is a fairly marked very diffuse increase in interstitial fibrous tissue and a moderate atrophy of the proximal convoluted tubules (fig. 3.13).

The histological changes in the kidney in renal vein thrombosis

Although the changes described by Rosenmann *et al.* (1968) of diffuse thickening of the glomerular basement membrane, leucocyte stasis, with tubular atrophy and interstitial fibrosis are present in a majority of cases, other cases may show very little change. It is also clear that changes present in the kidney progress with the passage of time.

Of the 2 cases with biopsies described here, 1 showed membranous thickening in the biopsy but no significant tubular or interstitial changes. In the autopsy specimen 7 years later, the glomerular changes had progressed and there was tubular atrophy and interstitial fibrosis. The other case did not even show membranous thickening in the first biopsy. The second biopsy, 12 months later, showed only membranous thickening with no definite tubular or interstitial changes whereas the autopsy specimen 1½ years after the second biopsy shows marked glomerular, tubular, and interstitial changes. It would seem from these cases that the histological changes may not be present in the early stages and may develop fairly slowly.

The margination of leukocytes was present in only 1 of the 4 cases, and in only 3 of the 7 cases analysed by Pollak *et al.* including Case 3 described here.

The relationship of renal vein thrombosis to the nephrotic syndrome

When as a result of the first biopsy studies of cases of nephrotic syndrome with renal vein thrombosis it was found that a majority of the cases had thickening of the glomerular basement membrane it was assumed that this thickening was also an effect of the venous thrombosis. Panner (1963) showed in 1 case that the electron microscope appearances were identical with those found in membranous nephropathy without renal vein thrombosis but it was still widely assumed that such changes could be produced by renal vein thrombosis.

In recent years opinion seems to be moving against this view. Ehrenreich and Churg (1968) in their series of 60 cases of membranous nephropathy had 10 autopsied cases and 5 of these had thrombosis of the main renal veins or their radicals. They accept such thrombosis as a complication of chronic membranous nephropathy. Bariéty *et al.* (1970) put forward the view that in such cases of membranous nephropathy (glomerulopathies extramembraneuses, G.E.M.) it is often impossible to say whether the thrombosis is a cause or result of the disease. Rosenmann *et al.* (1968) accept this view and comment on the fact that included in their series are a case of acute post-streptococcal glomerulonephritis and a case of diabetic nephropathy causing nephrotic syndrome in which renal vein thrombosis probably occurred as a consequence of the disease.

It has long been held by some authorities (e.g. Addis, 1948) that there is an increased tendency to venous thrombosis in the nephrotic syndrome. Recent studies of the coagulation mechanism in nephrotic syndrome (Kendall *et al.*, 1971) show elevated levels of plasma fibrinogen, factor V, combined VII, and X and VIII, mild thrombocytosis and accelerated thromboplastin regeneration and so support this clinical finding.

Such a thrombotic tendency would provide an explanation for the high incidence of renal vein thrombosis in nephrotic syndrome due to renal amyloidosis. The incidence in such cases in which a careful search is made at autopsy is 30 per cent (Milne, 1961). Clearly in these cases renal amyloidosis is not a consequence of the renal vein thrombosis.

Experimental renal vein constriction has been shown to produce nephrotic syndrome but only after constriction of one renal vein and removal of the contralateral kidney and then only in a proportion of the animals. Omae *et al.* (1958) produced severe proteinuria and hypercholesterolaemia in 8 of 41 rats so treated. Fisher *et al.* (1968) using a similar experimental procedure produced abnormal proteinuria, hyperlipidaemia and hypoproteinaemia in 47 per cent of rats. Fisher *et al.* (1968) examined the kidneys of these rats by electron microscopy. They found only loss of foot processes and other changes common to proteinuria of many different causes. They further examined with the electron microscope the glomeruli of 2 cases of nephrotic syndrome with renal vein thrombosis and 1 case of membranous nephropathy without renal thrombosis. They considered that these 3 cases showed changes in the glomeruli that were indistinguishable one from another and that these changes, the typical electron microscope appearances of membranous nephropathy were quite different from the changes found in their experimental animals. On this basis they were led to the view that the changes commonly found in the glomerular basement membrane in association with renal vein thrombosis are the primary condition and that the venous thrombosis is a consequence of the nephrotic syndrome produced by the glomerular lesion.

Accepting that renal vein thrombosis is most commonly a result of the nephrotic syndrome due either to membranous nephropathy or renal amyloidosis it nevertheless would seem highly probable that bilateral occlusion of the renal veins must produce some effect on renal function and structure. Constriction of the renal veins in the remaining kidney in experimental animals does produce proteinuria in 20 to 47 per cent of animals so that if renal vein thrombosis occurred in established nephrotic syndrome one would expect at least an increase in the proteinuria and it would seem likely that chronic venous obstruction might well produce interstitial oedema leading to fibrosis and also tubular atrophy.

In this context Case 3 described here is of interest as there was a clear history of trauma to the groin producing femoral vein thrombosis which then apparently spread up to involve the inferior vena cava and renal veins. Similar cases have been reported. Baird and Buchanan (1962) describe a case following post-operative thrombosis of the inferior vena cava. Proteinuria of 23 per day was found a month after the urine had been found to contain no protein.

It would be of great interest to examine with the electron microscope the glomeruli of such cases in which the renal vein thrombosis was clearly determined by some external cause. Presumably like the rats of Fisher *et al.* (1968) they would not show the appearances of membranous nephropathy.

Primary renal diseases

This group of cases is very mixed. It includes cases of many different types. However in recent years two important entities have been more clearly defined as a result of clinical studies based on renal biopsies. The nomenclature used by different groups of investigators unfortunately varies but clearly the diseases they are describing are the same. They are what I have previously referred to as 'minimal change' glomerulonephritis and membranous glomerulonephritis. The third group of cases are those with proliferative glomerulonephritis. Some progress has been made in defining separate entities in this group. This will be discussed in more detail in the next chapter.

'Minimal change' glomerulonephritis

This is the group of cases which although having marked proteinuria show no significant abnormality when the kidneys are examined by light microscopy. Such cases have been recognised for many years in autopsy material (Dunn, 1934) but unfortunately the nomenclature is still confused. In the United States it is commonly referred to as lipoid nephrosis (Pollak *et al.*, 1968; Forland and Spargo, 1969; Kawano *et al.*, 1971) but this term is unsatisfactory as the expression 'nephrosis' originally was introduced to describe a tubular lesion, but in these cases although the glomeruli appear normal by light microscopy changes are always demonstrable by electron microscopy. Furthermore the term has been used by Bell (1950) and Allen (1962) as a clinical term synonymous with nephrotic syndrome.

Unfortunately there is no entirely acceptable alternative. This difficulty was discussed at the Ciba symposium on renal biopsy (1961) and Hamburger pointed out the need for a term which says in one or two words 'optically normal glomeruli with fusion of the foot processes and slight epithelial changes on electron microscopic examination. This could be referred to as "minimal changes".' This is the term I will use as the best available.

The criteria for classifying a renal biopsy from a patient with nephrotic syndrome in this group are in the main negative ones. The glomeruli appear normal by light microscopy and in particular show no evidence of membranous or proliferative glomerulonephritis. Sometimes there is difficulty in deciding whether or not small focal areas of proliferation are present particularly at the centres of the lobules of the tuft. Slight degrees of epithelial cell proliferation are easier to detect as the epithelial cells generally become larger as well as increasing in number. It must, however, be remembered that the lesion in focal proliferative glomerulonephritis may be present in only a quarter of the glomeruli so they could be missed in a small biopsy with only a few glomeruli.

In most cases of 'minimal change' glomerulonephritis the renal biopsy appearances present little diagnostic difficulty. However in a significant minority the diagnosis depends on the assessment of very minor changes which might represent slight proliferation such as a few small groups of endothelial cells or a single capsular adhesion. These doubtful cases such as those for example in the Medical Research Council Study of prednisone in nephrotic syndrome (Black *et al.*, 1970) which were classified by one pathologist as 'minimal change' glomerulonephritis and by another pathologist as proliferative glomerulonephritis do differ from undoubted cases of 'minimal change' glomerulonephritis in that they do not respond to steroid therapy but they also differ from obvious proliferative glomerulonephritis in that they are much more likely to lose their proteinuria whether treated with steroids or not.

In this borderline between 'minimal change' glomerulonephritis and mild proliferative glomerulonephritis the usual subjective methods of assessment are somewhat unsatisfactory. It is possible that in the near future developments of modern morphometric methods may make this difficult distinction more certain.

Unfortunately two recent studies have produced apparently contradictory results. Kimmelstiel and his colleagues (Kawano *et al.*, 1971) in a series of 20 patients originally considered to have lipoid nephrosis made measurements of glomerular area and mesangial area and also counted the number of epithelial cell nuclei, endothelial cell nuclei, and mesangial cell nuclei. They found they were able to make a distinction between these cases and cases of proliferative glomerulonephritis. The two most important differences were in the mesangial area expressed as a percentage of the total glomerular area and the count of mesangial nuclei as a percentage of the total. They found in normals the mean percentage mesangial area was 7 per cent, in the cases of lipoid nephrosis it was 10·4 per cent and in the cases of proliferative glomerulonephritis it was 14·6 per cent. The figures for percentage of mesangial nuclei were normals 26 per cent, lipoid nephrosis 29·0 per cent and proliferative glomerulonephritis 42·4 per cent. On the basis of the percentage mesangial area they divided the presumed cases of lipoid nephrosis into two groups, one in which the percentage mesangial area was less than 10·7 per cent, and the other in which it was more than 10·7 per cent. Of the 11 cases in the first group detailed re-examination confirmed the diagnosis in 10 but in the second group of 9 cases, 3 were considered on re-examination to be proliferative glomerulonephritis, 1 was shown by electron microscopy to be membranous nephropathy, a further 3 were considered to be borderline cases and in only 2 cases was the diagnosis of lipoid nephrosis confirmed.

Kawano et al. (1971) concluded on the basis of this investigation that there is a non-inflammatory glomerular lesion which in most cases is associated with the clinical manifestations of the nephrotic syndrome.

However Wehner (1968) in a somewhat similar study found a definite increase in the mean number of nuclei per section of glomerulus from a mean of 29·1 in 1 μm sections of 20 normals to a mean of 37·6 in 20 cases of 'minimal change' glomerulonephritis. He found the increase to be mainly in mesangial cells. He concludes that 'minimal change' glomerulonephritis is therefore a mildly proliferative glomerulonephritis and suggests that it should be called acute membranous glomerulonephritis.

The reason for this discrepancy is not apparent. There are differences in the clinical cases. Those studied by Kawano et al. (1971) were children (mean age 2·7 years) and those studied by Wehner were older (mean age 19·6 years). Kawano et al. (1971) included as one of their diagnostic criteria a prompt response to steroid therapy. This would have excluded mild cases of proliferative glomerulonephritis.

There are also differences in the techniques. Wehner (1968) used 1 μm sections and made the counts directly down the microscope. Kawano et al. (1971) used 3 μm sections.

Case 5. Figures 3.14 and 3.15 show the kidney of a boy of 14 years. This was a biopsy including 23 glomeruli. It shows no significant histological change except hyaline droplet change in the tubules showing a striking distribution in small collections of closely grouped proximal convoluted tubules

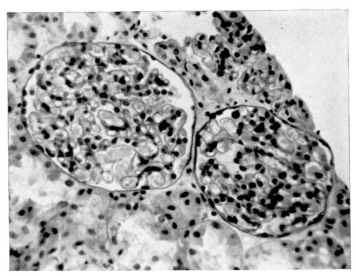

Fig. 3.14. Minimal change. Case 5. Two glomeruli showing no significant proliferative changes and no thickening of glomerular basement membrane. PAS × 250.

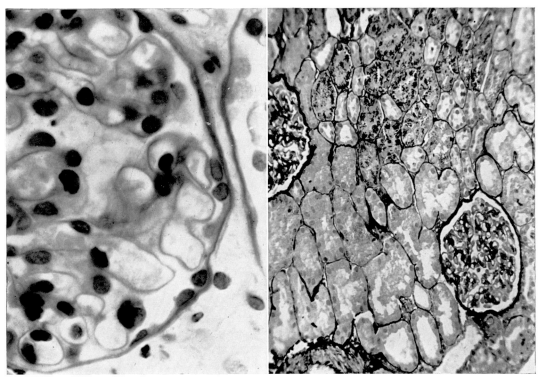

Fig. 3.15. Minimal change. Case 5. Higher power showing normal glomerular basement membrane. PAS × 900.

Fig. 3.16. Minimal change. Case 5. Cluster of proximal convoluted tubules containing prominent black staining hyaline droplets. PA silver × 200.

(fig. 3.16) presumably because protein reabsorption was occurring in only short lengths of tubules. At the time of the biopsy he had a serum albumin of 0·5 g/100 ml and a urinary protein loss of 10·2 g in 24 hours. He had had two previous attacks of nephrotic syndrome which had responded to steroid therapy. Fifteen months after the biopsy the serum albumin was 4·5 g/100 ml and there was no proteinuria. Nine years after the biopsy following 3 relapses when steroids were reduced he was off steroids and fully recovered with normal renal function and normal blood pressure.

In a number of cases second biopsies were performed so that the progress of the changes in the kidney could be examined. The following cases illustrate this.

Case 6. A woman of 39 who had nephrotic syndrome but had been treated with steroids before the biopsy. At the time of the biopsy there was no proteinuria. The serum albumin was 2·0 g/100 ml, and the creatinine clearance was 109 ml/min. The biopsy (fig. 3.17) shows no abnormality except striking dilatation of the glomerular capillaries. Her improvement was maintained and 23 months later at the time of the second biopsy there was again no proteinuria, the serum albumin was 4·4 g/100 ml and the creatinine clearance 119 ml/minute. The biopsy again showed no abnormality except dilatation of the glomerular capillaries (fig. 3.18).

Thirteen years after the first biopsy she is still on small doses of steroids. She is well, serum albumin 3·6 g/100 ml, creatinine clearance 120 ml/minute.

Case 7. A woman of 28 years at the time of the biopsy had a urinary protein loss of 9–11·4 g/24 hours, serum albumin 2·1–2·4 g/100 ml. The first biopsy (fig. 3.19) showed mainly normal glomeruli with one or two tufts showing a very doubtful increase in cellularity. Her proteinuria was reduced by the steroid therapy but initially was not abolished.

Twenty-three months later at the time of her second biopsy the 24-hour urinary protein loss was 5·8 g, serum albumin 2·83 g/100 ml and creatinine clearance 125 ml/minute. The biopsy again included normal glomeruli but also showed tufts with slight thickening at the centres of the lobules (fig. 3.20). This appearance resembles healing of a mild proliferative glomerulonephritis and raises the possibility that the case was initially wrongly classified.

However, 7 years after the initial biopsy she was well with no proteinuria, a serum albumin of 4·42 g/ 100 ml, and a creatinine clearance of 100 ml/minute.

Case 8. This girl developed nephrotic syndrome at the age of 15. Biopsy at this time (fig. 3.21) was classified as minimal change. Recent review of the section shows a doubtful increase in cellularity in a few glomeruli but there were small areas of undoubted proximal tubular damage. She was treated with steroids but failed to respond and died about 6 months after the onset. At post-mortem examination she was found to have suppurative pancreatitis. The kidneys (figs. 3.22 and 3.23) show an acute pyelonephritis with areas of fibrosis suggesting healing of previous episodes of acute pyelonephritis. There is

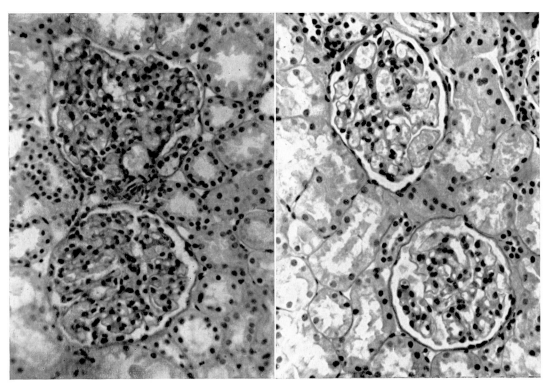

Fig. 3.17. Minimal change. Case 6. First biopsy. The only abnormality dilatation of capillaries in one glomerulus. PAS × 250.

Fig. 3.18. Minimal change. Case 6. Second biopsy 23 months after first. Only abnormality still dilatation of capillaries in one tuft. Tubules and interstitial tissue normal. PAS × 250.

moderate sclerosis of the glomeruli. Some of it may have resulted from healing of a previous proliferative glomerulonephritis, but the presence of pyelonephritis makes interpretation difficult.

Membranous nephropathy

This is now a clearly defined histological entity. The typical findings are of a thickening of the glomerular basement membrane (fig. 3.24) which affects it diffusely and equally within the tuft and in biopsies every glomerulus appears to be about equally involved. In post-mortem material Rich (1957) found that the changes were more advanced in the juxtamedullary glomeruli. I have not been convinced of this in biopsy material but this may be because cases are being studied earlier in their development.

Allen (1962) maintained that it is quite simple to recognise membranous glomerulonephritis in sections stained with haematoxylin and eosin. I think that if the basement membrane is markedly thickened it will be readily seen in haematoxylin and eosin sections. This is well seen in fig. 3.25. This renal biopsy is from a woman of 40 years of age (Case 9) who had proteinuria of 6·5–8·3 g/day, a serum albumin of 2·5 g/100 ml, and a creatinine clearance of 73 ml/min. However the thickening of the glomerular basement membrane is more obvious in the PAS preparations, particularly the higher power view (figs. 3.26 and 3.27). It is helpful in making the diagnosis to remember that the basement membrane thickening in membranous nephropathy is very diffuse and even in the peripheral capillaries of the tuft the basement membrane in each one will be thickened to about the same degree whereas in membranoproliferative glomerulonephritis the thickening is usually quite variable.

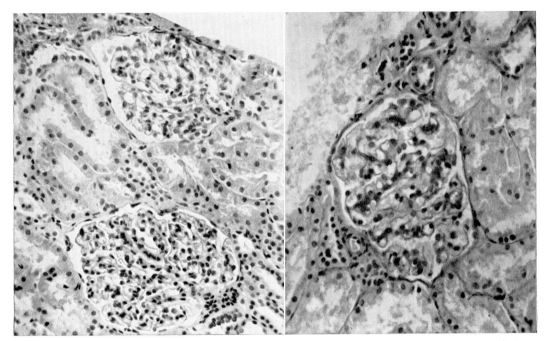

Fig. 3.19. Minimal change. Case 7. First biopsy. Doubtful centrilobular thickening and possibly increased cellularity. HE × 215.

Fig. 3.20. Minimal change. Case 7. Second biopsy 23 months after first. Slight hyaline thickening at centres of lobules. PAS × 250.

An important advance in the light microscope diagnosis of membranous nephropathy is the use of thin sections stained by the periodic acid silver methenamine method. Using the plastic embedding method described in the appendix it is fairly simple to cut 1·0 μm sections. When these sections are stained by the PA silver method the result is very striking and diagnostic. The inner portion of the basement membrane stains as a line but the outer portion stains irregularly producing the appearances of irregular bristles projecting from the membrane (fig. 3.28).

Five cases of membranous nephropathy have been examined in which 2 biopsies have been performed at intervals of from 7 to 57 months. In all except the case with an interval of only 7 months between the biopsies there was definite progression of the glomerular lesions.

This is the usual course of cases of membranous nephropathy. Although the progression of the disease may be very slow in the very considerable majority of cases it is inexorable.

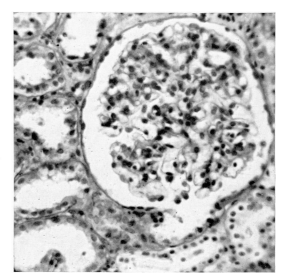

Fig. 3.21. Minimal change. Case 8. Glomerulus in biopsy showing slight endothelial cell proliferation. PAS × 250.

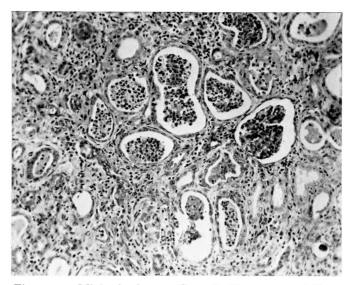

Fig. 3.22. Minimal change. Case 8. Post-mortem kidney. Active pyelonephritis. Cellular casts in dilated tubules. Marked interstitial fibrosis. PAS × 150.

It has recently been shown that with progression of the disease changes take place in the appearance of the glomeruli as seen in thin PA silver sections (Ehrenreich and Churg, 1968; Bariéty *et al.*, 1970). It can be seen with the electron microscope that the 'bristles' on the external surface of the basement membrane are extensions of the basement membrane projecting outward between subepithelial deposits which do not stain with the silver stain and hence are not seen by light microscopy. As the disease progresses the number of subepithelial deposits and the number of 'bristles' increases. Then the silver staining material extends circumferentially

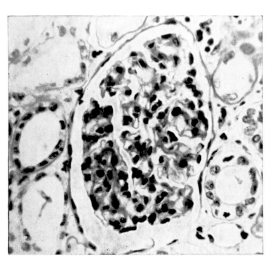

Fig. 3.23. Minimal change. Case 8. Post-mortem kidney. Golmerulus showing irregular mainly centrilobular thickening. PAS × 450.

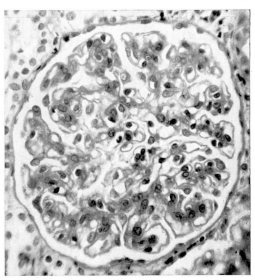

Fig. 3.24. Membranous nephropathy. Marked diffuse thickening of glomerular basement membrane. PAS × 435.

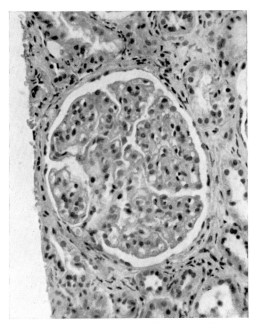

Fig. 3.25. Membranous nephropathy. Case 9. The glomerular tuft appears rather solid with reduced capillary lumens due to thickening of glomerular basement membrane. HE × 215.

from the tips of the 'bristles' surrounding the deposits and joins up the tips of the 'bristles' to form a pattern like the links of a chain. (Fig. 3.29.)

Remission of the clinical manifestations of the nephrotic syndrome with resolution of the structural changes in the glomerulus are rare but a few well documented cases have now been

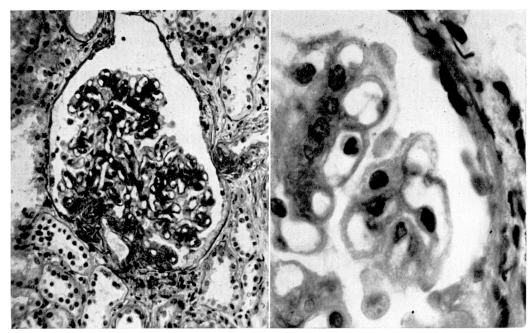

Fig. 3.26. Membranous nephropathy. Case 9. The thickening of the glomerular basement membrane is rather more evident. PAS × 215.

Fig. 3.27. Membranous nephropathy. Case 9. Thickening of glomerular basement membrane strikingly evident at this magnification. PAS × 900.

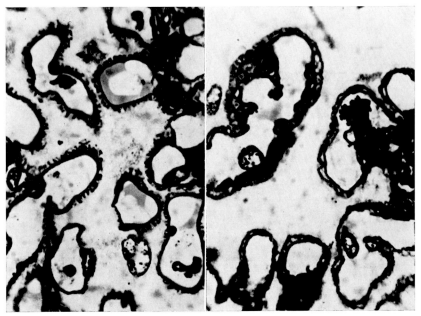

Fig. 3.28. Membranous nephropathy. 1 μm plastic embedded section. Striking 'bristles' on external surface of glomerular basement membrane. PA silver × 920.

Fig. 3.29. Membranous nephropathy. 1 μm plastic embedded section. Late stage showing link of bristles to form an irregular chain. PA silver × 920.

reported. Bariéty *et al.* (1968) describe 2 patients shown by biopsy to have membranous nephropathy in whom after $2\frac{1}{2}$ and 4 years of remission further biopsy showed a considerable reduction in the lesion. Forland and Spargo (1969) described a similar favourable course in 1 of their 19 cases. Renal biopsy in the third year of a clinical remission showing striking regression of previously marked membranous changes.

Case 10. Fig. 3.30 and fig. 3.31 are two biopsies taken at an interval of 2 years from a man aged 21 at the time of the first biopsy when the urinary protein loss was 18–22 g daily, serum albumin 1·15 g/100 ml and creatinine clearance 68 ml/minute. Clearly during the 2 years there has been considerable progression of the glomerular lesion. At the time of the second biopsy the proteinuria was 4·7 g daily, the serum albumin 2·04 g/100 ml, and the creatinine clearance 58 ml per minute.

He has survived 10 years after the first biopsy but still has proteinuria of 6·5 g/24 hours, serum albumin 2·7 g/100 ml, serum creatinine 2·8 mg/100 ml, and a creatinine clearance of 30 ml/minute.

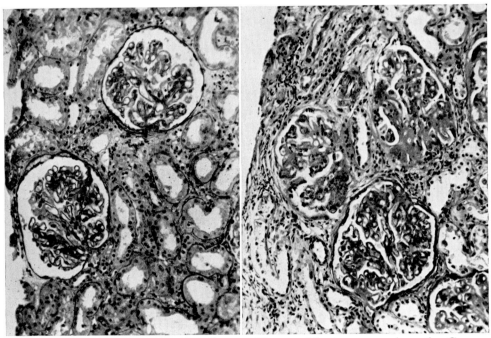

Fig. 3.30. Membranous nephropathy. Case 10. First biopsy. Two tufts showing quite marked diffuse thickening of the glomerular basement membrane. The tubules are almost normal and there is only very slight interstitial fibrosis. PAS × 150.

Fig. 3.31. Membranous nephropathy. Case 10. Second biopsy 2 years after first. Three tufts showing marked irregular sclerosis. PAS × 150.

Case 11. The other two biopsies (figs. 3.32 and 3.33) illustrated are from a woman of 42 years. At the time of her first biopsy the daily urinary protein loss was 6·3–10·3 g, serum albumin 1·7 g/100 ml and creatinine clearance 53 ml/minute. The second biopsy, taken 57 months after the first, shows marked irregular hyalinisation of glomeruli. Clinically, she was surprisingly well but her blood pressure was 220/124 mm having been 170/100 mm when first seen. The daily urinary protein loss was still 6·0 g, serum albumin 2·49 g/100 ml and creatinine clearance 46 ml/minute.

Proliferative glomerulonephritis

In recent years there has been some progress in our understanding of this group of diseases. There has been considerable progress in our knowledge of possible mechanisms of

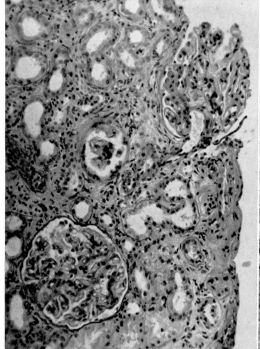

Fig. 3.32. Membranous nephropathy. Case 11. First biopsy. Moderate diffuse thickening of glomerular basement membrane. Diffuse interstitial fibrosis. PAS × 150.

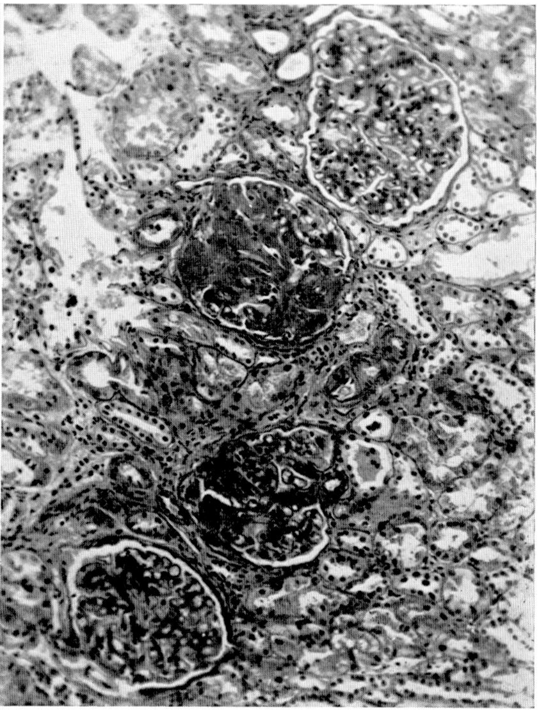

Fig. 3.33. Membranous nephropathy. Case 11. Second biopsy 57 months after first. Marked sclerosis of 2 middle tufts. PAS × 135.

pathogenesis. This has been admirably summarised by Dixon (1968). There has also been some advance in our knowledge of the various entities included within this heterogeneous group, mainly as a result of the clear recognition of the entity now most commonly known as membrano-proliferative glomerulonephritis. Despite this it is clear that this group still includes a number of ill-defined entities, the nature of which will become clearly defined by further careful clinico-pathological studies. In this chapter they are classified on a simple morphological basis. The development of the various lesions and their relationship to one another will be discussed in more detail in the next chapter.

Predominantly endothelial cell proliferation

Figure 3.34 shows a typical example with an obvious diffuse increase in cellularity due to an endothelial cell proliferation with no evidence of epithelial cell proliferation. There are also small numbers of polymorphs present appearing as small darkly staining irregularly shaped nuclei. At the time of taking the biopsy this 26-year-old woman (Case 12) had proteinuria of 9–12 g daily, serum albumin 1·7 g/100 ml. The further history is considered later (Case 6 in Chapter 4).

In some cases of endothelial cell proliferation glomerulonephritis in addition to the cellular proliferation there is also formation of a good deal of fibrillar material. Such cases have given rise to some confusion and difficulty. In haematoxylin- and eosin-stained sections they have sometimes been mistaken for membranous nephropathy. Such a case is illustrated in figs. 3.35 and 3.36. Figure 3.35 of a section stained with haematoxylin and eosin is very similar to fig. 3.25

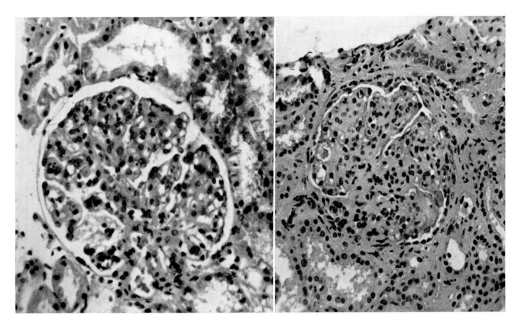

Fig. 3.34. Proliferative glomerulonephritis. Case 12. Marked increase in cellularity of tuft due mainly to endothelial cell proliferation but with also a small number of polymorphs. HE × 250.

Fig. 3.35. Proliferative glomerulonephritis. Endothelial cell proliferation with rather diffuse thickening. Compare with fig. 3.25. HE × 215.

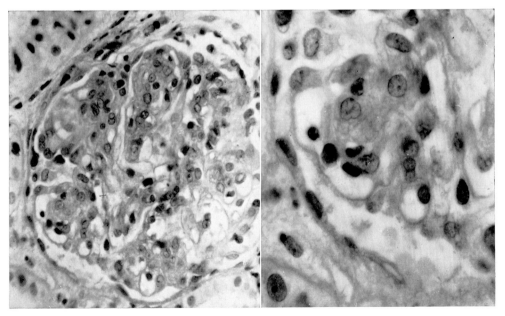

Fig. 3.36. Proliferative glomerulonephritis. Same case as fig. 3.35. Thickening mainly centrilobular with cellular proliferation in some areas. Note few capillary loops with basement membrane not thickened. PAS × 450.

Fig. 3.37. Proliferative glomerulonephritis. Same case as fig. 3.35 and 3.36. Peripheral glomerular basement membrane not thickened. Compare with fig. 3.27. × 900.

of a case of membranous nephropathy similarly stained. The condition illustrated in figs. 3.35–3.37 is membranoproliferative glomerulonephritis. Until recently there was often confusion between this entity and membranous nephropathy resulting in the use of such expressions as mixed membranous and proliferative glomerulonephritis implying that the condition might be membranous nephropathy with a superimposed proliferative glomerulonephritis. It is now clear that this is not so and that membranoproliferative glomerulonephritis and membranous nephropathy are two entirely separate and readily diagnosable conditions. They can often be distinguished in PAS stained sections particularly if attention is paid to the basement membrane in the peripheral glomerular capillaries. It is consistently thickening in membranous nephropathy but in membranoproliferative glomerulonephritis its thickness often varies considerably. The distinction can be more readily made in thin (1·0 μm) sections stained by the periodic acid methenamine silver method. As has already been shown sections of membranous nephropathy stained by this method show a very typical appearance consisting of 'bristles' on the external surface of the glomerular basement membrane (fig. 3.28). In membranoproliferative glomerulonephritis the thickening is on the inner surface of the original glomerular basement membrane and is produced by a thin layer of mesangial cell cytoplasm and newly formed fibrils which often produce the characteristic appearance of a double-layered basement membrane (fig. 3.38).

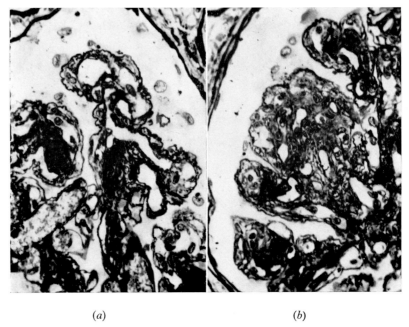

(a)   (b)

Fig. 3.38. Membranoproliferative glomerulonephritis. Marked thickening at centres of lobules. Typical double basement membrane in several capillaries. PA silver × 370.

Lobular glomerulonephritis

The characteristic appearance is seen in fig. 3.39. It is now clear that there is no evidence for the suggestion that this type of nephritis develops from membranous nephropathy and that it is probably a variant of membranoproliferative glomerulonephritis but this will be discussed in detail in the next chapter.

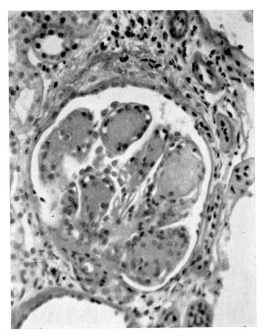

Fig. 3.39. Lobular glomerulonephritis. Striking round acellular masses at the centres of the lobules. PAS × 250.

Focal glomerulonephritis

In this type of nephritis small proliferative lesions are present in a proportion of the glomerular tufts whilst the remaining tufts appear normal. In the affected tufts the lesions are confined to one or two lobules (fig. 3.40). As with the other proliferative glomerular lesions the clinical manifestations are very varied. In the series of Heptinstall and Joekes (1961) 10 of the 31 cases

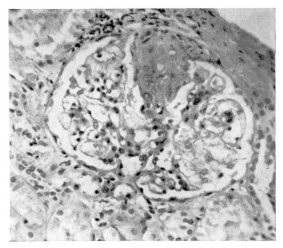

Fig. 3.40. Focal glomerulonephritis. Case 13. A very cellular solid proliferative lesion sharply confined to one lobule. PAS × 150.

presented with the nephrotic syndrome. Two cases had both nephrotic syndrome and Henoch–Schonlein syndrome.

Case 13. A man of 31 complained of nausea and tiredness for 2 weeks, swelling of his ankles for 24 hours and a gain of 10 lb in weight. His blood pressure was 160/80, serum urea 33 mg/100 ml, serum albumin 2 g/100 ml and a daily protein loss of 5–6 g. He had a petechial rash and a clinical diagnosis of Henoch-Schonlein purpura was made. He made a good recovery. Six years after the biopsy his renal function was normal, creatinine clearance 127 ml/min, no proteinuria and normal B.P.

Proliferative glomerulonephritis with crescents

In a proportion of cases of proliferative glomerulonephritis with nephrotic syndrome quite large crescents are found, a somewhat surprising finding in view of the commonly held view that such histological findings are associated with the clinical syndrome of so-called type I nephritis. Figure 3.41 illustrates such a case with a large cellular crescent almost filling Bowman's space. The patient (case 14) was a man of 58 years who, at about the time of biopsy, had a urinary

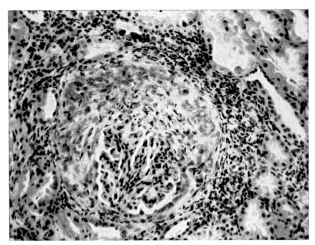

Fig. 3.41. Proliferative glomerulonephritis with crescents. Case 14. A cellular crescent almost completely obliterates Bowman's space. HE × 150.

protein loss of 5–15 g daily, a serum albumin of 1·7–2·0 g and a creatinine clearance of 23–50 ml per minute. There was marked oedema of the legs, back and scrotum. The blood pressure was 210/110 mm. He improved slightly but the proteinuria persisted at about 3–6 g daily. He died in uraemia 2½ years after the biopsy.

The prognosis in nephrotic syndrome

The first observations combining assessment by renal biopsy with study of the response to treatment appear to be those of Bjørnboe *et al.* (1952). They studied 6 patients. Two in whom the biopsies showed few or no definite histological changes responded favourably to ACTH. The 4 who did not respond had shown pronounced changes on renal biopsy.

In recent years the prognosis of the different forms of primary renal disease causing nephrotic syndrome and their response to steroid therapy have been more clearly defined. The only controlled trial of steroid therapy is that organised by the British Medical Research Council (Black *et al.*, 1970). In this trial a total of 125 patients were studied, 31 with 'minimal change' glomerulonephritis, 19 with membranous nephropathy, and 75 with proliferative glomerulonephritis.

Patients were allocated randomly to a prednisone and nonprednisone treatment group. The results showed that in 'minimal change' glomerulonephritis prednisone had a rapid and striking effect in reducing the proteinuria but was without significant effect on membranous nephropathy or proliferative glomerulonephritis.

Several other groups of investigators have described similar results. Forland and Spargo (1969) summarise their experience by saying that 60 per cent of lipoid nephrosis responds to steroids but such a response is infrequent in membranous nephropathy. They further found that the mortality in 'minimal change' glomerulonephritis was less than 10 per cent but in membranous nephropathy it was about 50 per cent. Hopper *et al.* (1970) obtained a cure (defined as freedom from proteinuria for 1 year or longer) in 74 per cent of cases of 'minimal change' glomerulonephritis. Pollak *et al.* (1968) compared 21 patients with 'minimal change' glomerulonephritis (lipoid nephrosis) with 21 patients with membranous nephropathy and confirmed the much better prognosis and the good response to steroid therapy in 'minimal change' glomerulonephritis.

Difficulties in diagnosis

Renal biopsy remains the most reliable method of determining the cause of the nephrotic syndrome and so in many cases enabling an accurate prognosis to be made. There are however published accounts of small numbers of cases of 'minimal change' glomerulonephritis which followed an unfavourable course (McGovern, 1964; Hayslett *et al.*, 1969). Such cases are quite exceptional and many of them I suspect are wrongly diagnosed. Certainly some of the published illustrations of such cases seem to me to show mild proliferative changes.

Most cases of 'minimal change' glomerulonephritis and membranous nephropathy can be readily diagnosed but occasional cases give rise to difficulty. These difficulties are of two sorts. One is to distinguish between 'minimal change' glomerulonephritis and mild proliferative glomerulonephritis, the other is to distinguish between 'minimal change' glomerulonephritis and early membranous nephropathy.

In resolving the first difficulty one would hope that some form of nuclear count might be helpful. As the work of Kawano *et al.* (1971) and Wehner (1968) shows there are difficulties which need to be resolved before this method becomes a practical possibility. Until such a method becomes available I think that in making a diagnosis of 'minimal change' glomerulonephritis even the slightest evidence of proliferation should be considered to exclude the case from this category. This viewpoint is supported by the experience of the British Medical Research Council steroid trial (Black *et al.*, 1970). In this trial the category of very mild proliferative glomerulonephritis (diagnosed independently by one pathologist as proliferative glomerulonephritis and by another as 'minimal change' glomerulonephritis) behaved differently from definite 'minimal change' glomerulonephritis in that they did not respond to steroid therapy but they also differed from definite proliferative glomerulonephritis (agreed by both pathologists) in that regardless of whether or not they were given steroids they were much more likely to lose their proteinuria.

The distinction between 'minimal change' glomerulonephritis and established membranous nephropathy can usually be readily made using PAS stained sections. Difficulty only arises in the early cases of membranous nephropathy when the basement membrane thickening may be slight. Such cases may easily be mistakenly diagnosed as 'minimal change' glomerulonephritis and such mistakes account for some of the reported cases of 'minimal change' glomerulonephritis which follow an unfavourable course and in which the histological changes of membranous nephropathy are then said to develop.

Many of these mistakes can be avoided by preparing 1 μm sections stained by the PA silver technique. Whether all errors can be avoided remains uncertain. Ehrenreich and Churg (1968) in their study of 67 biopsies from 60 patients in which 50 biopsies were studied by electron microscopy came to the conclusion that in making the diagnosis a good PA silver stain on a 2–3 μm section was usually an adequate substitute for electron microscopy. However Bariéty *et al.* (1970) in a similar combined light and electron microscopy study claim that in the very early stages of membranous nephropathy changes may be found on electron microscopy whilst the light microscope appearances are still normal.

REFERENCES

ADDIS, T. (1948). *Glomerular Nephritis.* Macmillan, New York, p. 216.

ALLEN, A. C. (1962). *The Kidney* (2nd edition) Churchill, London, pp. 248, 308.

BAIRD, W. L. and BUCHANAN, D. P. (1962). *Amer. J. Med.* **32**, 128.

BARCLAY, G. P. T., CAMERON, J. M. and LOUGHRIDGE, L. W. (1960). *Quart. J. Med.* **29**, 137.

BARIÉTY, J., DRUET, PH., SAMARCQ, P. and LAGRUE, G. (1969). *J. Urol. Nephrol.* **75**, 627.

BELL, E. T. (1950). *Renal Disease.* Henry Kimpton, London. pp. 206, 230.

BERGER, J., DE MONTERA, H. and GALLE, P. (1961). *Arch. Anat. path.* **9**, 313.

BERGSTRAND, A. and BUCHT, H. (1961). *J. Path. Bact.* **81**, 495.

BJØRNBOE, M., BRUN, C., GORMSEN, H., IVERSEN, P. and RAASCHOU, F. (1952). *Acta. med. scand. suppl.* **266**, 249.

BLACK, D. A. K., ROSE, G. and BREWER, D. B. (1970). *Brit. med. J.*, **3**, 421.

BLAINEY, J. D., BREWER, D. B., HARDWICKE, J. and SOOTHILL, J. F. (1960). *Quart. J. Med.* **29**, 235.

BLAINEY, J. D., HARDWICKE, J. and WHITFIELD, A. G. W. (1954). *Lancet* **ii**, 1208.

CARONE, F. A. and EPSTEIN, F. H. (1960). *Amer. J. Med.* **29**, 539.

CHURG, J., HABIB, RENEE and WHITE, R. H. R. (1970). *Lancet* **i**, 1299.

DIXON, F. J. (1968). *Amer. J. Med.* **44**, 493.

DUNN, J. S. (1934). *J. Path. Bact.* **39**, 1.

EARLE, D. P., JR. (1960). *Proc. Ann. Conf. Neph. Synd.* **12**, 272. Ed. METCOFF, J. Nat. Kidney Dist. Found., New York.

EHRENREICH, T. and CHURG, J. (1968). *Path. Ann.* **3**, 145.

FISHER, E. R., SHARKEY, D., PARDO, V. and VUZERSKI, V. (1968). *Lab. Invest.* **18**, 689.

FOLLI, G., POLLAK, V. E., REID, R. T. W., PIRANI, C. L. and KARK, R. M. (1958). *Ann. intern. Med.* **49**, 775.

FORLAND, M. and SPARGO, B. H. (1969). *Nephron* **6**, 498.

GEER, J. C., STRONG, J. P., MCGILL, H. C. and MUSLOW, I. (1958). *Lab. Invest.* **7**, 554.

HASSON, J., BERKMAN, J. I., PARKER, J. G. and RIFKIN, H. (1957). *Ann. intern. Med.* **47**, 493.

HAYSLETT, J. P., KRASSNER, L. S., BENSCH, K. G., KASHGARIAN, M. and EPSTEIN, F. H. (1969). *New. Engl. J. Med.* **281**, 181.

HEPTINSTALL, R. H. and JOEKES, A. M. (1961). *Renal Biopsy.* Ciba Foundation Symposium. Churchill, London, p. 194.

HOBBS, J. R. and MORGAN, A. D. (1963). *J. Path. Bact.* **86**, 437.

HOPPER, J., JR., RYAN, P., LEE, J. C. and ROSEMAN, W. (1970). *Med. (Balt.)* **49**, 321.

KARK, R. M., PIRANI, C. L., POLLAK, V. E., MUEHRCKE, R. C. and BLAINEY, J. D. (1958). *Ann. intern. Med.* **49**, 751.

KAWANO, K., WENZL, J., MCCOY, J., PORCH, J. and KIMMELSTIEL, P. (1971). *Lab. Invest.* **24**, 499.

KENDALL, A. G., LOHMANN, R. C. and DOSSETOR, J. B. (1971). *Arch. intern. Med.* **127**, 1021.

LAWRENCE, J. R., POLLAK, V. E., PIRANI, C. L. and KARK, R. M. (1963). *Med. (Balt.)* **42**, 1.

MCCLUSKEY, R. T. (1971). *J. exp. Med.* **134**, 242S.

MCGOVERN, V. J. (1964). *Aust. Ann. Med.* **13**, 306.

MAXWELL, M., ADAMS, D., BERNSTEIN, D. and KLEEMAN, C. (1970). *Proc. Ann. Conf. Neph. Synd.* **12**, 261. Ed. METCOFF, J. Nat. Kidney Dis. Found., New York.

MILNE, M.D. (1961). *Renal Biopsy.* Ciba Foundation Symposium. Churchill, London, p. 363.

MOVAT, H. Z. (1960). *Arch. Path.* **69**, 323.

NESSON, H. R., SPROUL, E., RELMAN, A. S. and SCHWARTZ, W. B. (1963). *Ann. intern. Med.* **58**, 269.

OMAE, T., MASSON, G. M. C. and CORCORAN, A. C. (1958). *Proc. Soc. exp. Biol. (N.Y.)* **97**, 821.

PANNER, B. (1963). *Arch. Path.* **76**, 303.

POLLAK, V. E., KARK, R. M., PIRANI, C. L., SHAFTER, H. A. and MUEHRCKE, R. C. (1956). *Amer. J. Med.* **21**, 496.

POLLAK, V. E., ROSEN, S., PIRANI, C. L., MUEHRCKE, R. C. and KARK, R. M. (1968). *Ann. intern. Med.* **69**, 1171.

RICH, A. R. (1957). *Bull. Johns Hopk. Hosp.* **100**, 173.

RICHTER, G. W. (1954). *Amer. J. Path.* **30**, 239.

ROSENBLATT, M. B. (1936). *Arch. intern. Med.* **57**, 562.

ROSENMANN, E., POLLAK, V. E. and PIRANI, C. L. (1968). *Med. (Balt.)* **47**, 269

SPENCER, A. G. (1959). *Postgrad. med. J.* **35**, 613.

SQUIRE, J. R., HARDWICKE, J. and SOOTHILL, J. F. (1962). *Renal Disease.* Ed. BLACK, D. A. K. Blackwell, Oxford, p. 216.

VERNIER, R. L., WORTHEN, H. G. and GOOD, R. A. (1961). *J. Pediat.* **58**, 620.

WEHNER, H. (1968). *Verh. dtsch. Ges. Path.* **52**, 288.

4

Glomerulonephritis

It is still not possible to devise a complete and consistent classification of glomerulonephritis but over recent years there has been a steady growth in knowledge of the various entities encompassed within this term. This has come about mainly by careful studies of biopsy material combined with detailed studies of the clinical manifestations and life histories of the various clinical forms of glomerulonephritis so that correlations have been established between various histological appearances and clinical entities. Evidence of this process in action has been the almost simultaneous recognition of the detailed life history of membranous nephropathy in France (Bariéty *et al.*, 1969) and in the United States (Ehrenreich and Churg, 1968) and also the widespread acceptance of membranoproliferative glomerulonephritis as an entity with characteristic histological, immunofluorescent, and clinical manifestations (Cameron *et al.*, 1970; Herdman *et al.*, 1970; Bariéty *et al.*, 1971; Mandalenakis *et al.*, 1971).

These advances are the result of the empirical approach of carefully defining what is seen in the biopsy and correlating it with the clinical findings. I will therefore continue to consider the cases of glomerulonephritis in groups based on simple morphological criteria. The first group, glomerulonephritis with predominantly endothelial cell proliferation is probably most usually

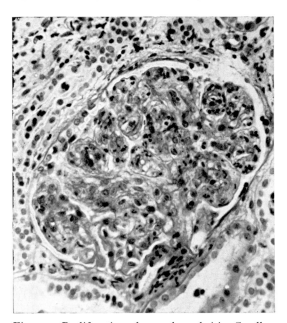

Fig. 4.1. Proliferative glomerulonephritis. Swollen cellular glomerulus due mainly to severe endothelial cell proliferation. Small numbers of polymorphs present. Capillaries obliterated. PAS × 250.

post-streptococcal glomerulonephritis. I consider lobular glomerulonephritis with this first group as it is possible that it develops from it. Membranoproliferative glomerulonephritis is also probably related to lobular glomerulonephritis and in both there is probably more mesangial cell proliferation than endothelial cell. Focal glomerulonephritis appears to be a distinct morphological entity. Lupus nephritis is probably an aetiological entity but may show any of a wide range of morphological changes.

The final group, glomerulonephritis with crescents, is considered in two grades of severity.

Endothelial cell proliferative glomerulonephritis

Following the excellent work of Jennings and Earle (1961) it seems likely that this is post-streptococcal in origin. The glomeruli are swollen and much more cellular than normal. This is evident from the great increase in nuclei present. These are mainly large pale-staining nuclei, but amongst them can be seen the small lobed darkly staining nuclei of polymorphs. Often in the more severe cases as in fig. 4.1 it is difficult to see any capillary lumens. However in less severe cases capillary lumens can be seen (fig. 4.2). The tendency for cells to be grouped at the centres of the lobules is also evident. PA silver preparations show a large amount of very fine fibre in these areas (figs. 4.3, 4.4) and sometimes the peripheral basement membrane appears double but even so the fibres are still very fine (fig. 4.5).

Case 1. This patient was a boy of 13 who 4 months before the biopsy complained of swelling of the face, abdomen and limbs with dark urine. His B.P. was 198/110, blood urea 120 mg/100 ml, and antistreptolysin titre 833 units. At the time of the biopsy he had generalised oedema, huge ascites, the 24-hour urinary protein loss was 5–10 g, serum albumin 1·51 g/100 ml, blood urea 27 mg/100 ml and creatinine clearance 34 ml per minute. He made a fairly good recovery. Four months later his B.P. was 140/80, urinary protein 0·17 g/100 ml, serum albumin 3·0 g/100 ml, blood urea 23 mg/100 ml, and creatinine clearance 40 ml per min. Three years after the onset of the illness, the B.P. was 136/80, blood urea 27 mg/100 ml, urinary protein 0·1 g/100 ml, serum albumin 4·5 g/100 ml and creatinine clearance 71 ml per minute.

However following this his renal function deteriorated and dialysis commenced 5 years after the biopsy. Eight years after the biopsy he died of haemorrhage from his A–V fistula which he disconnected.

The extent of the endothelial cell proliferation in these cases varies considerably. In the biopsy illustrated in figs. 4.6 and 4.7 there are only quite small focal areas of cellular proliferation.

Case 2. The patient was a man of 25 who 4 months before the biopsy was diagnosed clinically as suffering from acute nephritis. This illness settled with bed rest but haematuria and proteinuria later recurred. At the time of the biopsy the B.P. was 158/105, 24-hour urinary protein loss was 2·9–10·9 g, serum albumin 3·6–3·4 g/100 ml, blood urea 22 mg/100 ml, and creatinine clearance 123 ml/minute. The proteinuria persisted but at a considerably reduced rate. Two and a half years later his blood pressure, blood urea and serum albumin were all normal. Ten years after the biopsy his full recovery is still maintained.

The other extreme of severity is illustrated in fig. 4.8 (Case 3). The very cellular tuft shows some tendency to lobulation. There is also a very small amount of epithelial cell proliferation. Figures 4.9 and 4.10 show that the cellular proliferation has obliterated the capillary lumens. There is a good deal of fibre formation at the centres of the lobules but the peripheral basement membrane is still quite thin.

Case 3. This biopsy is from a boy of 16 whose illness began with a sore throat followed 10–12 days later by haematuria and oedema. At the time of the biopsy some weeks after the onset he had a B.P. of 150/90, 24-hour urinary protein loss of 12–20 g, serum albumin 1·8 g/100 ml, creatinine clearance of 49 ml/minute and blood urea 40 mg/100 ml. He improved slightly but following another throat infection rapidly deteriorated. Four weeks after the biopsy following this sudden deterioration he was grossly oedematous, B.P. 200/130. His renal function became progressively impaired, his blood urea steadily rose from 375 mg to 596 mg/100 ml and he died of renal failure 10 weeks after the biopsy.

Fig. 4.2.   Fig. 4.5.

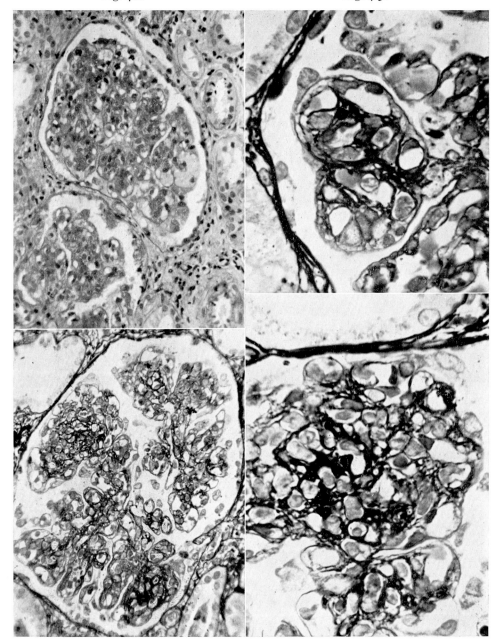

Fig. 4.3.   Fig. 4.4.

Fig. 4.2. Proliferative glomerulonephritis. Case 1. Extensive endothelial cell proliferation but capillary lumens still visible. PAS × 250.

Fig. 4.3. Proliferative glomerulonephritis. Case 1. PA silver × 370.

Fig. 4.4. Proliferative glomerulonephritis. Case 1. Marked cellular proliferation in centrilobular area with much fine fibre formation. PA silver × 900.

Fig. 4.5. Proliferative glomerulonephritis. Case 1. Peripheral lobule. Capillary lumen patent. Formation of fine fibre producing appearance of double basement membrane. PA silver × 900.

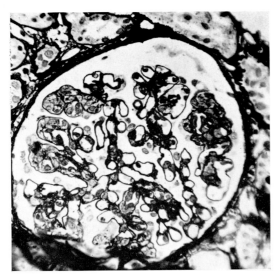

Fig. 4.6. Proliferative glomerulonephritis. Case 2. Only a few capillary loops are obliterated by endothelial cell proliferation. PA silver × 370.

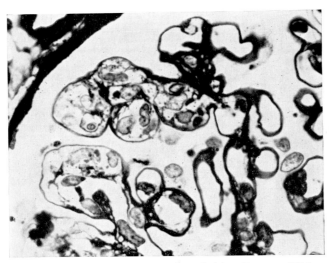

Fig. 4.7. Proliferative glomerulonephritis. Case 2. Higher power of capillaries occluded by proliferated endothelial cells. PA silver × 900.

In 4 cases 2 biopsies have been performed at intervals varying from 5 to 22 months. They all show similar changes consisting mainly of a tendency for the tufts to become more lobulated and for thickening to occur at the centres of the lobules.

Case 4. A girl 18 years of age at the time of the biopsy had suffered an attack of acute nephritis when 13. She had made a good recovery with ACTH and steroids. At the age of 18 following skin testing she developed oedema and another attack of nephritis developed. At the time of the first biopsy (fig. 4.11) the creatinine clearance was 140 ml/minute, the 24-hour urinary protein loss 10·7 g, and the serum albumin 2·58 g/100 ml. Her condition did not respond to prednisone but with hydroxychloroquine the

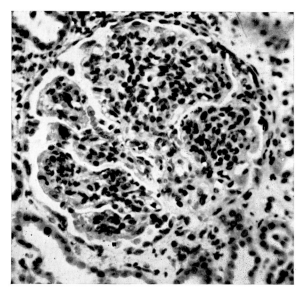

Fig. 4.8. Proliferative glomerulonephritis. Case 3. Extreme endothelial cell proliferation. Slight epithelial cell proliferation. Rather lobulated tuft. PAS × 250.

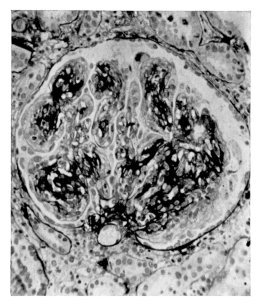

Fig. 4.9. Proliferative glomerulonephritis. Case 3. PAS × 235.

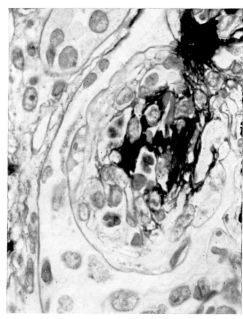

Fig. 4.10. Proliferative glomerulonephritis. Case 3. Peripheral lobule of glomerulus. Extreme endothelial cell proliferation obliterating capillary lumen. Peripheral basement membrane still very thin. PA silver × 900.

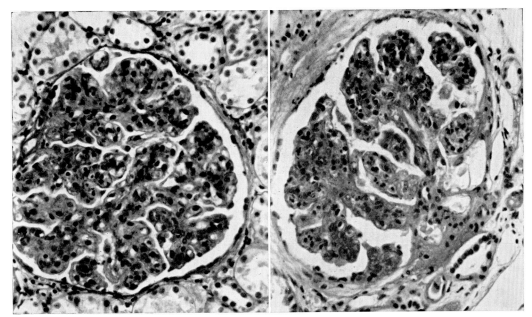

Fig. 4.11. Proliferative glomerulonephritis. Case 4. First biopsy. Marked endothelial cell proliferation with moderate numbers of polymorphs. PAS × 250.

Fig. 4.12. Proliferative glomerulonephritis. Case 4. Second biopsy 22 months after first. Still marked endothelial cell proliferation and many polymorphs. Tuft lobulated. PAS × 250.

proteinuria fell. The second biopsy (fig. 4.12) was performed 22 months after the first. At this time the creatinine clearance was 33 ml/minute, the 24-hour urinary protein loss 8·1 g and the serum albumin 2·26 g/100 ml.

The glomeruli still appear rather cellular with proliferated endothelial cells and polymorphs. The tufts are now rather lobulated.

She died of chronic renal failure 3 years and 9 months after the first biopsy. Her terminal serum creatinine was 18 mg/100 ml.

Case 5. A man of 37 first complained of puffiness of the face, dysuria, oliguria and dark urine. There was slight oedema.

The first biopsy was performed 2 months after the onset of the illness when 24-hour urinary protein loss was 7–10 g, serum albumin 1·9 g/100 ml and the blood urea 270 mg/100 ml. The tufts are enlarged and cellular as a result of endothelial cell proliferation obliterating the capillaries. There are no obvious polymorphs (fig. 4.13).

The second biopsy 5 months later shows considerable resolution, but with quite definite thickening at the centres of the lobules (fig. 4.14). At this time the daily urinary protein loss was 1·5–2·5 g, serum albumin 2·74 g/100 ml, and the blood urea 44 mg/100 ml.

Sixteen months later he had no symptoms, the serum albumin was 3·8 g/100 ml but his B.P. was 180/120.

Eleven years after the first biopsy he was maintaining a full recovery, serum creatinine 1·3 mg/100 ml, blood urea 24 mg/100 ml, proteinuria less than 1 g/day, B.P. 150/100.

The thickening that develops at the centres of the lobules varies considerably in degree so that in the more severe cases it comes to resemble chronic lobular glomerulonephritis. There is no evidence as to whether this depends on the severity of the initial attack or possibly on recurrent attacks.

Case 6 shows progression of the glomerular changes with quite marked centrilobular thickening in the second biopsy. This woman of 23 had an attack of acute nephritis at the age of 19 when she had oedema

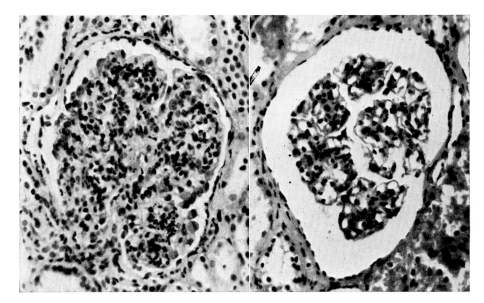

Fig. 4.13. Proliferative glomerulonephritis. Case 5. First biopsy. Cellular swollen glomerulus. Proliferative endothelial cells obliterated capillaries. HE × 250.

Fig. 4.14. Proliferative glomerulonephritis. Case 5. Second biopsy 5 months after first. Glomeruli much less cellular. Cells grouped in centres of lobules. Capillary lumens present. PAS × 250.

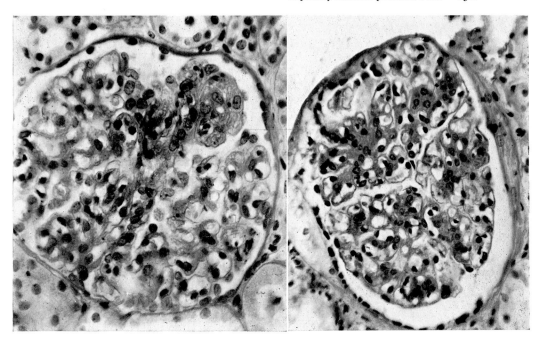

Fig. 4.15. Proliferative glomerulonephritis. Case 6. First biopsy. Endothelial cell proliferation and small numbers of polymorphs. PAS × 450.

Fig. 4.16. Proliferative glomerulonephritis. Case 6. Second biopsy 9 months after first. Striking grouping of cells at centres of lobules about areas of quite marked hyaline thickening. PAS × 370.

of the legs and face, a daily urinary protein loss of 3 g and a serum albumin of 3·6 g/100 ml. She made a good recovery but the condition recurred and at the time of the first biopsy (fig. 4.15) the daily urinary protein was 9–12 g, serum albumin 1·7 g/100 ml and blood urea 27 mg/100 ml. Nine months later at the time of the second biopsy the daily urinary protein loss was 3·4 g, serum albumin 2·36 g/100 ml, blood urea 56 mg/100 ml and the B.P. was 140/90. The second biopsy shows quite marked thickening at the centres of the lobules (fig. 4.16). Despite this, renal function has remained good. Three years and four months after the first biopsy the serum albumin was 3·7 g/100 ml, blood urea 32 mg/100 ml, creatinine clearance 133 ml/minute and B.P. 146/90.

Rather surprisingly this good progress has been maintained. Nine years after the first biopsy there is no proteinuria, B.P. is normal, serum creatinine 1·1 mg/100 ml and blood urea 27 mg/100 ml.

Discussion

This group of cases, which appears to me to be a fairly homogeneous one, corresponds in the initial stages and in its subsequent development to what Jennings and Earle (1961) have shown to be post-streptococcal glomerulonephritis.

They describe a series of 36 patients in whom glomerulonephritis was proved in each case to have followed group A haemolytic streptococcal infection. The histological changes found were primarily glomerular. The most characteristic changes consisted of endothelial cell proliferation which in the early stages was diffuse but later became more focal and located in the 'stalks' of each glomerular lobule. There was also exudation characterised by an increased number of polymorphs within the capillary loops. Epithelial crescents were present in 13 of the 36 patients.

The cases varied considerably in severity. In 7 cases the disease was so slight that the diagnosis depended mainly on laboratory findings. One patient became anuric and died 32 days after the onset. In 13 of the remaining 35 the nephritis had not healed at the last follow up which in 6 cases was more than 12 months. (Healing was defined as permanent disappearance of proteinuria, at least 4 protein-free urines obtained over several weeks. Persistence of proteinuria for a year or more after onset was considered reasonably good evidence of chronicity.)

The presenting symptoms generally consisted of haematuria, proteinuria, oedema, hypertension and nitrogen retention. There was a fairly good correlation between the estimated severity of the glomerular lesion and nitrogen retention, maximum diastolic pressure and the presence of oedema. Only 1 case of the 36 developed nephrotic syndrome.

A study by Lawrence et al. (1963) confirms the histological findings in post-streptococcal glomerulonephritis. They examined renal biopsies from a series of 84 adult cases of nephrotic syndrome and found 9 cases of post-streptococcal glomerulonephritis and a further 13 probable cases.

McCluskey and Baldwin (1963) also examined a series of 25 cases of acute glomerulonephritis and found that 10 developed the nephrotic syndrome. (Proteinuria resulting in a decrease of serum albumin to less than 3 g/100 ml).

The histological findings in post-streptococcal glomerulonephritis and the changes found in the glomeruli as they resolve have been confirmed recently by several groups of workers (Dodge et al., 1968; Salle et al., 1968).

Prognosis

There are now several studies of the natural history of post-streptococcal glomerulonephritis with detailed bacteriological and biopsy data.

The older studies were of the clinical and bacteriological aspects of the disease and in general gave a very good prognosis. Thus Ellis (1942) gave the recovery rate of acute glomerulonephritis (Ellis Type I) as 80–90 per cent. Rammelkamp (1953) also considers that the prognosis is very good. In fact he doubts whether chronic glomerulonephritis is ever the result of a previous attack of post-streptococcal glomerulonephritis.

The prognosis in biopsy series has not been as good as this. In the series of Jennings and Earle (1961) of 36 cases, 22 were considered to have recovered, 13 had not healed and had been followed up for periods ranging from 4 to 46 months, and there was 1 death from anuria. Of the 25 cases described by McCluskey and Baldwin (1963) 5 died, 6 recovered and 14 were still active at the time of report. Kushner *et al.* (1961) found clinical healing in 22 of 29 cases. However in some cases healed apparently clinically there was still histological evidence of activity. There were, in fact, 14 cases with either clinical or histological evidence of chronicity.

It seems clear that the major reason for the reported differences in prognosis is in the selection of cases. Thus Rammelkamp's cases mainly arose during convalescence from type 12 streptococcal pharyngitis. The diagnosis was based on mild proteinuria and microscopic haematuria. Very few of the patients had oedema, hypertension or impairment of renal function. In most biopsy series almost all the cases had obvious clinical manifestations except in the series of Jennings and Earle (1961) in 7 of whose 36 patients the diagnosis depended mainly on laboratory findings.

In the 3 biopsy series there was a general relationship between the severity of the histological changes and the clinical manifestations including the subsequent healing. There were occasional exceptions to this. One case in the series of Jennings and Earle had no hypertension or oedema and only mild impairment of renal function yet there was definite glomerular hypercellularity and the disease failed to heal.

Jennings and Earle (1961) thought that chronic changes developed as a result of the progression of the changes induced in the acute attack. They did not think that repeated exacerbations were important in the progression of acute to chronic glomerulonephritis.

McCluskey and Baldwin (1936) agree with this. They believe that the intensity of the disease process reaches its peak early and then slowly regresses. They think that true exacerbations with the reappearance of exudative and proliferative changes occur rarely if at all. Their combined experiences are considerable and their suggestion probably correct, but it is worthwhile noting that Case 4 of this chapter after a history of an attack of acute nephritis at the age of 13 suffered another episode of acute nephritis at the age of 18 and still had evidence of active proliferative changes with polymorphs in a second biopsy taken 22 months after the second attack. Case 6 also had a history of an attack of acute nephritis four years before the first biopsy yet showed active proliferative changes in the glomeruli.

The results of recent biopsy studies of post-streptococcal glomerulonephritis (Dodge *et al.*, 1968; Salle *et al.*, 1968) in general agree with the previous studies although the results have been somewhat better but it is clear that careful follow up will demonstrate that clinical return to complete normality may be slow and resolution of the histological changes even slower. Dodge *et al.* (1968) studied a series of 44 children with typical post-streptococcal glomerulonephritis. Six (14 per cent) had histopathological evidence of pre-existing renal disease. Twenty of the remaining 38 were observed for periods of up to 2 years or more. In 45 per cent there was clinical evidence of non-healing. Sixteen patients had renal biopsies 2 years after onset and 50 per cent of these had histological evidence of non-healing. The patients whose lesions healed were significantly younger at the onset of their disease and also showed higher maximum ASO titres than those whose lesions did not heal. The study by Salle *et al.* (1968) includes only 10 children but they were observed over a period of 31 months with repeated renal biopsies. Second biopsies were performed at intervals of between 6 and 13 months. In only 3 cases was the proliferation considerably reduced. In 5 cases it persisted unchanged. Third biopsies were performed in 5 children between 15 and 24 months after onset. In 3 cases there was considerable regression of the histological changes but there was still present some proliferation of endo-thelial cells and mesangial cells with enlargement of the mesangium. In one case the proliferative changes remained identical with those in the previous two biopsies. Fourth biopsies were per-formed 31 months after the onset of the disease in 2 children. In one case there were present only small amounts of segmental and focal hyalinisation. The other case, which had shown persistence of proliferative changes in all the previous 3 biopsies showed the same degree of proliferative changes in the fourth biopsy. Salle *et al.* (1968) concluded from these findings that the histological changes persist often for a considerable time after apparent clinical and functional resolution. This is confirmed by Treser *et al.* (1969). They studied 23 children who had apparently recovered completely from post-streptococcal glomerulonephritis as judged by the fact that they were asymptomatic and had normal blood pressures, normal urea clearances and 3 consecutive normal Addis counts. All patients were biopsied between 1 and 3 years after the onset of the acute disease and only 4 of the 23 were found to be normal. The remaining 19 had segmental mesangial lesions and varying amounts of gamma-globulin and complement were demonstrated in the glomeruli by immunofluorescence. Subsequent biopsies showed fur-ther resolution of the glomerular lesions in 16 cases, but in 3 cases there was morphological evidence of progression of the glomerular lesion and complement and gamma-globulin could still be demonstrated by immunofluorescence. They came to the conclusion that the presence or absence of complement or gamma-globulin was the most reliable indicator of whether the glomerular damage would progress or resolve.

Membranoproliferative glomerulonephritis and lobular glomerulonephritis

These two morphological entities have been incompletely described separately and together over many years (for reference to earlier studies see Mandalenakis *et al.*, 1971). Amongst the first papers describing the association between the histological changes and low levels of serum complement were those of West *et al.* (1965) and Gotoff *et al.* (1965). It is only recently that there has been widespread acceptance of membranoproliferative glomerulonephritis as a histological entity with a characteristic clinical picture and course and often with characteristic immuno-logical manifestations (Cameron *et al.*, 1970; Herdman *et al.*, 1970; Bariéty *et al.*, 1971; Mandalenakis *et al.*, 1971).

The histological appearances of the glomeruli in membranoproliferative glomerulonephritis are typical. They are increased in size, there is proliferation of endothelial cells and mesangial cells, there is an increase in eosinophilic and PAS-positive fibrillar material at the centres of the lobules and the basement membrane of the glomerular capillaries (fig. 4.17) appears irregularly thickened. However the appearances can readily be distinguished from membranous nephro-pathy by the evidence of proliferation but most readily and unequivocally by the appearance of the glomerular basement membrane as seen in thin PA silver sections. As has been previously illustrated in membranous nephropathy (fig. 3.28) there are on the external surface of the glo-merular basement membrane many short little 'bristles' which in the later stages of the disease join up to form a pattern like the links of a chain.

In membranoproliferative glomerulonephritis the original glomerular basement membrane can still be seen not to be thickened and with a smooth external surface. The thickening is internal to it and in PA silver sections is seen to consist of a pale layer and often then a second layer of black-staining thin basement membrane producing a double layered glomerular base-ment membrane (fig. 4.18). It can be seen with the electron microscope that the pale middle layer, in fact, consists of cytoplasm of proliferated mesangial cells that have moved around beneath the endothelium to encircle the glomerular capillaries.

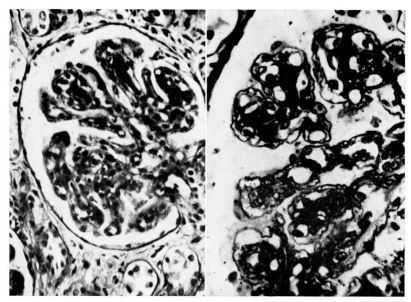

Fig. 4.17. Membranoproliferative glomerulonephritis. Widespread irregular mesangial thickening and variable thickening of peripheral basement membrane. HE × 230.

Fig. 4.18. Membranoproliferative glomerulonephritis. 1 μm plastic embedded section. Marked mesangial thickening. Several capillaries have a double-layered basement membrane. PA silver × 370.

The disease may follow a very slow indolent course (Herdman *et al.*, 1970) marked by episodes of gross haematuria and oedema frequently associated with anaemia and hypertension. One or other clinical manifestation may predominate so that Cameron *et al.* (1970) divided their 50 cases into 4 groups according to their modes of onset. Twenty-three presented with nephrotic syndrome, 12 with symptomless proteinuria, 12 with an acute nephritic syndrome and 3 with recurrent haematuria.

A striking immunological finding is that in a majority of cases there is a marked reduction in the C3 component of serum complement (β_1C globulin). Cameron *et al.* (1970) found reduced levels initially in 68 per cent of their cases and in a further 16 per cent the levels subsequently fell.

Immunofluorescent studies of renal biopsies have further shown that β_1C globulin is deposited along the glomerular basement membrane. Herdman *et al.* (1970) found such deposition in all of 43 biopsy specimens from 20 of their patients and similar findings are described by Bariéty *et al.* (1971) and by Mandalenakis *et al.* (1971).

Although the prognosis for recovery is very poor the clinical course of the disease may be very prolonged. Most patients survive for 10 years and a reasonable number for at least 15 years and for many years renal function may be surprisingly well maintained despite very severe histological changes.

Lobular glomerulonephritis

Lobular glomerulonephritis was recognised as a histological entity some years ago before the entity of membranoproliferative glomerulonephritis was defined. Allen (1962) originally suggested that lobular glomerulonephritis developed from membranous nephropathy. This is clearly wrong. The current evidence strongly favours the view that lobular glomerulonephritis and membranoproliferative glomerulonephritis are manifestations of the same process which consists of proliferation mainly of mesangial cells with irregular formation of fibrillar basement membrane-like material but that in lobular glomerulonephritis this material accumulates in acellular nodules at the centres of the lobules pushing the cells and capillaries to the periphery (figs. 4.19 and 4.20).

Case 7. This renal biopsy was taken from a young girl of 18. (It is also illustrated in fig. 3.39). During pregnancy she was found to have proteinuria of about 1·5 g/day. The serum albumin was 3·3 g/100 ml, B.P. 150/90 and creatinine clearance 67 ml/minute.

Four years after the biopsy the B.P. was 130/90 and the blood urea 39 mg/100 ml.

Ten years after the biopsy she was clinically well with a normal B.P. but still had proteinuria of 6·0 g/day and a serum albumin of 2·5 g/100 ml. Twelve years after the biopsy she refused to attend the Renal Clinic. She was reported to be still well but with 'heavy proteinuria'.

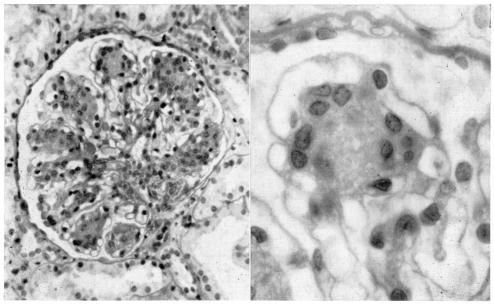

Fig. 4.19. Lobular glomerulonephritis. Case 7. Marked hyaline thickening at the centres of the lobules with grouping of cells about them. PAS × 250.

Fig. 4.20. Lobular glomerulonephritis. Case 7. Higher power of fig. 4.19 showing peripheral basement membrane not thickened. PAS × 900.

Cameron *et al.* (1970) divided their 50 cases of membranoproliferative glomerulonephritis into a lobular and non-lobular group. They found that those classified as lobular were generally younger and more often had an onset of the acute nephritic type than the non-lobular group and that although the groups could not be clearly separated on their complement levels all the eight patients in their series with persistently normal levels of complement were in the non-lobular group. However their final conclusion was that the lobular and non-lobular forms are not separate entities but are variants of the same condition. Both Bariéty *et al.* (1971) and Mandalenakis *et al.* (1971) agree with this conclusion.

There is some evidence that lobular glomerulonephritis may follow an attack of acute glomerulonephritis. Thus Berger *et al.* (1961) describe 10 cases of chronic lobular glomerulonephritis with nephrotic syndrome. In 4 cases there was a history highly suggestive of preceding acute glomerulonephritis. They suggest that chronic lobular glomerulonephritis results from hyalinisation following an endocapillary proliferative glomerulonephritis centred about the centrilobular areas. In 1 case they were able to follow the development of the nodules in 2 successive biopsies and in autopsy material.

Lawrence *et al.* (1963) support this idea and also illustrate the development of lobular glomerulonephritis in serial biopsies.

Despite this suggestive evidence recent studies of membranoproliferative glomerulonephritis have provided no evidence of its aetiology.

Focal glomerulonephritis

Focal glomerulonephritis is the condition in which acute lesions, generally proliferative in character, but sometimes showing necrosis, occur in only a proportion of glomeruli and within the affected glomeruli involve only one or two lobules, the remainder of the tuft appearing normal. The striking contrast between the affected and unaffected areas within a single glomerular tuft is well shown in fig. 3.40. Some authors attach importance to the fact that the changes affect only a proportion of glomeruli, sparing others. The striking distribution of the changes within individual glomerular tufts seems to me to be much more important.

Case 8. A man of 27 at the time of the first biopsy had suffered an attack of renal colic in the preceding year. At the time of the biopsy he had the nephrotic syndrome with heavy proteinuria 16–30 g daily, serum albumin 0·68 g/100 ml, B.P. 125/80 and creatinine clearance 144 ml/minute.

The biopsy (fig. 4.21) shows active proliferative lesions affecting quite small areas of several tufts. There were many tufts that appear normal. It is commonly assumed that such tufts are completely normal. With such small lesions limited to a part of the tuft obviously many sections cut through an affected glomerulus would not include the lesion. The second biopsy taken 2 years and 11 months after the first shows small hyaline acellular areas in many tufts, presumably the result of healing of the acute lesions (fig. 4.22). Despite this the proteinuria has continued.

Four years and three months after the first biopsy the daily urinary protein loss was 5·5 g. The creatinine clearance was however well maintained at 130 ml/minute.

Twelve years after the first biopsy he is well but still has proteinuria of 2 g/day, and serum albumin 2·9 g/100 ml. His creatinine clearance is 150 ml/min.

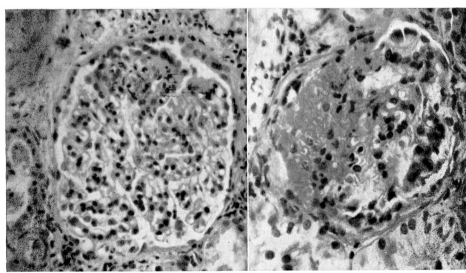

Fig. 4.21. Focal glomerulonephritis. Case 8. First biopsy. A small area at periphery of tuft showing endothelial and epithelial proliferation with also a few polymorphs. HE × 250.

Fig. 4.22. Focal glomerulonephritis. Case 8. Second biopsy 35 months after first. Hyaline acellular areas in tuft presumably acute lesions healed with steroid therapy. PAS × 450.

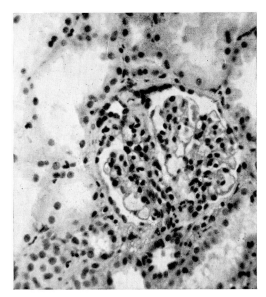

Fig. 4.23. Focal glomerulonephritis. Case 9. Biopsy specimen. Lesion at periphery of tuft with small area of adhesion. HE × 250.

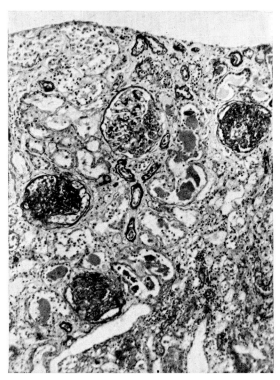

Fig. 4.24. Focal glomerulonephritis. Case 9. Autopsy specimen. Severe sclerosis of several glomeruli. PAS × 100.

In the series of Heptinstall and Joekes (1961) of the 31 patients, 13 made a complete recovery, 12 however showed evidence of a persisting renal lesion and 4 of these had a persisting or progressive renal functional impairment. These 4 cases had extensive lesions on biopsy.

An unfavourable outcome is illustrated in the following case.

Case 9. A young man of 19 presented with nephrotic syndrome. Biopsy at the time (fig. 4.23) showed focal lesions in many glomeruli. Many of them took the form of small localised areas of adhesion covered by plump epithelial cells. The appearances suggest that the lesions had been present for some time and were healing. All the lesions in the biopsy appear about the same age.

He remained under treatment for 5 years ultimately developing hypertension, B.P. 200/145 and uraemia, the final urea was 750 mg per 100 ml.

Post-mortem examination showed the kidneys to be reduced in size (combined weight 230 g) with irregularly granular surfaces.

Histologically the kidneys show a severe chronic glomerulonephritis (fig. 4.24) with complete sclerosis of many glomeruli. There is a good deal of tubular atrophy and interstitial fibrosis.

Discussion

Focal glomerulonephritis occurs in association with several diseases so the clinical manifestations are very variable. The form in which it was first recognised was probably the focal embolic glomerulonephritis of subacute bacterial endocarditis. In these circumstances the clinical manifestations are mainly those of the cardiac lesion. The renal lesions of polyarteritis nodosa and Henoch–Schonlein purpura may also present the same histological picture though in both conditions the glomerular lesions are often more diffuse with striking crescents.

In most cases of focal glomerulonephritis however there is no evidence of any cause. Bates *et al.* (1957) described an outbreak of acute nephritis following pharyngitis which was shown not to be streptococcal.

Compared with post-streptococcal glomerulonephritis there was a shorter latent period between infection and the onset of nephritis, greater haematuria, less hypertension and oedema and less renal functional impairment. The glomerular damage was much milder and more focally distributed than post-streptococcal glomerulonephritis. It seems possible that some cases of focal glomerulonephritis may have a non-streptococcal infective cause.

Disseminated lupus erythematosus

It is difficult for anyone to add to the excellent study of Muehrcke *et al.* (1957) of a series of 33 patients suffering from disseminated lupus erythematosus; 25 of these patients had renal complications, mild in 10, severe in 12. They emphasise the pleomorphic nature of the lesions found and conclude that with the exception of haematoxyphil bodies there is no single histological finding which can be considered pathognomonic of the disease. In addition to haematoxyphil bodies they found 'wire looping' of the glomerular basement membrane, fibrinoid change, local and focal necrosis of glomerular tufts, hyaline thrombi and clumping and proliferation of endothelial cells. Although no single histological finding is diagnostic the diagnosis was relatively easy in many cases as several histological features occurred together. Thus the combination of 'wire looping', focal necrosis, fibrinoid and haematoxyphil bodies was considered diagnostic.

My experience has been limited to a small number of cases but even these showed a wide variety of changes.

Case 10. A girl of 19 had a generalised arthritis 3 years previously. L.E. cells were demonstrated. She now has nephrotic syndrome.

A biopsy shows a moderate diffuse thickening of the glomerular basement membrane affecting every glomeruli with quite marked but rather patchy proliferation of endothelial cells (fig. 4.25). There is no 'wire looping', no focal necrosis and no haematoxyphil bodies. The thickened basement membrane contains no fibrinoid.

Case 11. A 40-year-old man complained of dark, scanty urine appearing the day after he developed a sore throat after having been vaguely unwell for about 2 months. He had haematuria, proteinuria (2–4 g daily), uraemia (blood urea 104 mg/100 ml), a creatinine clearance varying from 45 to 66 ml/minute and a blood pressure of 160/100. A clinical diagnosis of lupus erythematosus was made but no L.E. cells were found.

Renal biopsy shows a very active proliferative glomerulonephritis with striking rather focal endothelial cell proliferation with numerous polymorphs in the glomerular capillaries (fig. 4.26).

He was treated with large doses of steroid and improved considerably. Four years later his blood urea was 40 mg/100 ml, creatinine clearance 102 ml/minute but he still had a proteinuria of 2·6 g daily and a B.P. of 160/100.

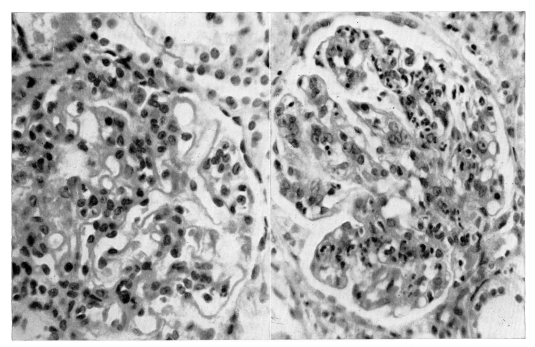

Fig. 4.25. Lupus nephritis. Case 10. Marked endothelial cell proliferation. Cells grouped at centres of lobules. Marked diffuse thickening of glomerular basement membrane. PAS × 450.

Fig. 4.26. Lupus nephritis. Case 11. Striking endothelial cell proliferation. Numerous polymorphs in capillaries. HE × 450.

Ten years after the biopsy he was clinically well and working full time. B.P. 150/100, serum creatinine 1·3 mg/100 ml, blood urea 45 mg/100 ml, proteinuria 30 mg/100 ml. Four years before this last assessment he had quite a bad relapse when the dose of steroids was reduced. When full dosage was resumed he recovered.

'Wire looping' occurs in a variety of conditions, malignant hypertension, scleroderma, dermatomyositis amongst others. It is however conspicuous in cases of disseminated lupus erythematosus. It consists of a thickening of the glomerular basement membrane which stains brightly pink with eosin and is often sharply limited to a few capillary loops. It stains positively with fibrin stains and with PAS (fig. 4.27).

The PA silver method produces a striking appearance of a paler smooth mass inside a thin black staining basement membrane (fig. 4.28). This biopsy is from another case in which a

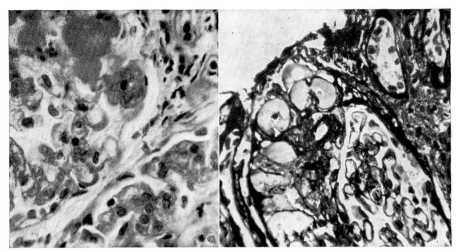

Fig. 4.27. Lupus nephritis. 'Wire looping'. Marked PAS positive thickening of glomerular basement membrane. Affected loops sharply localised. Thickening follows outline of loop. PAS × 450.

Fig. 4.28. Lupus nephritis. 'Wire looping'. Severely affected loops filled with smooth paler staining material with thin black basement membrane about it. PA silver × 450.

clinical diagnosis of disseminated lupus erythematosus was not supported by the finding of L.E. cells.

Glomerulonephritis with crescents

Epithelial crescents are commonly considered to be typical of the subacute stage of glomerulonephritis. However many cases of post-streptococcal glomerulonephritis never show crescents at any stage of the disease.

In other cases, many of them certainly not post-streptococcal, crescents are a striking feature being present in every tuft.

Case 12. A man of 42 developed a staphylococcal empyema following excision of a cyst of lung. Haematuria then developed with a blood urea of 103 mg/100 ml, proteinuria of 6 g/day, a blood pressure which varied from 120/80 to 155/100 mm Hg and a creatinine clearance of 26 ml/minute. His condition improved fairly rapidly on steroid therapy. Three months after the acute onset the haematuria was much diminished, the urine protein was 4·7 g daily, blood urea 53 mg/100 ml, and the creatinine clearance 42 ml/minute. After a further 2 months there was almost no significant haematuria, the creatinine clearance was 95 ml/minute, B.P. 160/100 and urinary protein 4·9 g per day.

At this time he suffered an upper respiratory infection and a quite marked increase in the haematuria occurred, but the proteinuria remained at about the same level 5·2 g per day. A renal biopsy was now performed 6 months after the onset. It shows a severe lesion with fibrosing crescents in many glomeruli and sharply demarcated areas of interstitial fibrosis including atrophic tubules (fig. 4.29).

In the succeeding months his renal function deteriorated, creatinine clearances falling to levels of 37–40 ml/minute.

Fourteen months after the onset he improved rapidly over a period of 2 months, creatinine clearances increasing to 180–190 ml/minute, proteinuria eventually falling to a trace. A second biopsy was performed at this time. It shows a surprising degree of resolution of the changes previously seen. Many glomeruli are normal. Others show areas of hyalinisation (figs. 4.30 and 4.31) that in some glomeruli replace the whole tuft. This type of hyalinisation appears to be particularly prominent in acute lesions resolving as a result of steroid therapy, as in this case. There is surprisingly little fibrosis in some areas.

Since this biopsy his condition has fluctuated somewhat but 6 years after the onset he had only a trace of protein in his urine, and a creatinine clearance of 110 ml per minute.

Twelve years after the first biopsy he is well with no proteinuria, serum creatinine 1·2 mg/100 ml, creatinine clearance 94 ml/minute and a normal B.P.

A small number of cases of glomerulonephritis develop severe oliguria or anuria very early in the disease. They show dramatic histological changes with very large cellular crescents completely obliterating Bowman's space. The prognosis is exceedingly grave. Even though the patients may be kept alive by haemodialysis the damage to the glomeruli is so severe that there seems no prospect of them ever regaining function.

Case 13. A man of 44 developed anuria after a very short history of haematuria and malaise which followed a sore throat. He was admitted to the General Hospital, Birmingham, anuric with a blood urea of 400 mg/100 ml. Haemodialysis was performed the day after admission. Four days after admission

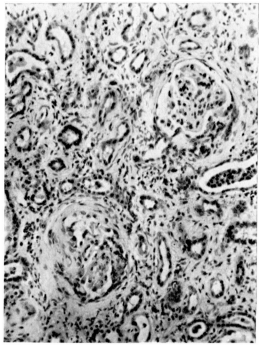

Fig. 4.29. Glomerulonephritis with crescents. Case 12. First biopsy. Two glomeruli with fibro-epithelial crescents. Marked interstitial fibrosis separating atrophic tubules. HE × 150.

a renal biopsy was performed. Bowman's space is completely filled by large cellular crescents (fig. 4.32). As can be well seen in the PA silver preparation the crescents at this stage contain no fibres. They consist of cells only (fig. 4.33). The urine flow never again exceeded 10 ml a day. A second biopsy was performed 6 weeks after the first. In some glomeruli the epithelial crescents have shrunk away slightly from Bowman's capsule leaving a small space (fig. 4.34). In haematoxylin and eosin stained sections it is difficult to separate tuft and epithelial crescent. This can readily be done in PA silver preparations which also show a good deal of connective tissue fibre within the crescent (fig. 4.35).

A total of 16 haemodialyses were performed. Death occurred as a result of a rapidly progressive peripheral neuritis 4 months after onset. The post-mortem kidneys show almost a complete destruction of every glomerulus by mature fibrous tissue. In PAS stained sections the rather shrunken glomerular tufts can be recognised staining more deeply than the fibrous tissue filling Bowman's space (fig. 4.36). The basement membrane of Bowman's capsule can still be recognised. In some cases the fibrous tissue can be seen extending into the proximal convoluted tubules (fig. 4.37).

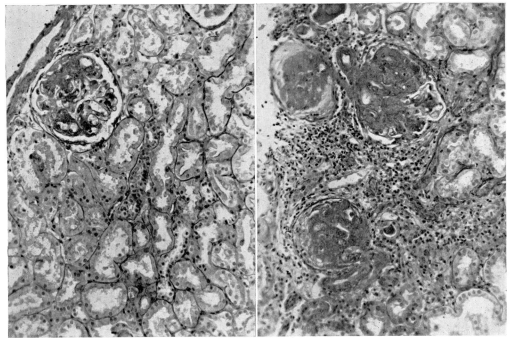

Fig. 4.30. Glomerulonephritis with crescents. Case 12. Second biopsy 14 months after first. Glomerulus showing irregular areas of hyalinisation. Normal tubules with no interstitial fibrosis. PAS × 150.

Fig. 4.31. Glomerulonephritis with crescents. Case 12. Second biopsy 14 months after first. Three severely sclerosed glomeruli with interstitial fibrosis and lymphocytic infiltration.

Some of these cases have also shown either in the biopsy or at autopsy acute necrotising arterial lesions.

Case 14. A man of 26 about 6 months before the onset of his terminal illness had an attack of right-sided abdominal pain diagnosed as renal colic. At this time the blood urea was 22 mg/100 ml. He recovered after 4 days in hospital. Following discharge he had several similar attacks each lasting a day. He was eventually re-admitted to hospital after an attack in which he vomited. Two days after admission he became anuric. He was transferred to the General Hospital, Birmingham, where he was dialysed 4 times. No urine was passed and he died of a cerebral haemorrhage, a month after the onset of the last illness.

A biopsy performed 10 days after onset of anuria shows extremely cellular crescents completely filling Bowman's space (fig. 4.38). It is impossible to separate tuft and crescent but the basement membrane of Bowman's capsule can still be seen as a thin line. As in many of these cases the proximal convoluted tubules are lined by rather flat cells suggesting regeneration after damage (fig. 4.39). (Figure 8.12 is taken from another similar case.)

At autopsy there was a necrotising arteriolitis of many arterioles in the kidney but none were found in any other organs.

The classification and diagnosis of glomerulonephritis

As our knowledge of the aetiology of glomerulonephritis remains incomplete the classification of glomerulonephritis also remains incomplete. However the classification as it exists is important as the different entities that can currently be defined have different prognoses and responses to treatment.

Post-streptococcal glomerulonephritis

This is the type of nephritis in which the aetiological role of a specific infection is most clearly established and there is very good evidence that the glomerular damage results from

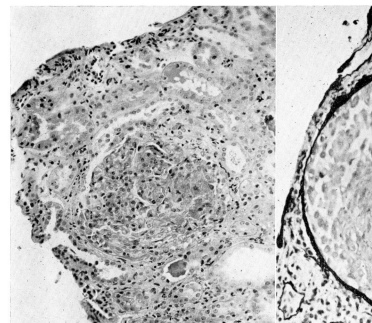

Fig. 4.32. Glomerulonephritis with crescents. Case 13. First biopsy. Bowman's space is obliterated by a large cellular crescent. PAS × 150.

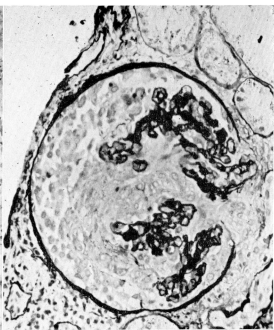

Fig. 4.33. Glomerulonephritis with crescents. Case 13. First biopsy. It can be seen that the crescent consists entirely of cells with no fibres. PA silver × 250.

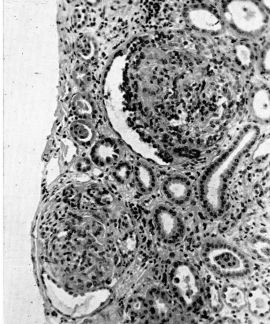

Fig. 4.34. Glomerulonephritis with crescents. Case 13. Second biopsy 6 weeks after first. Crescents now slightly shrunken. HvG × 150.

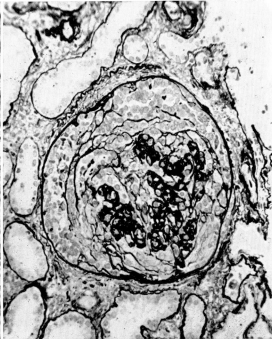

Fig. 4.35. Glomerulonephritis with crescents. Case 13. Second biopsy 6 weeks after first. A good deal of fine fibre now present in crescent. PA silver × 250.

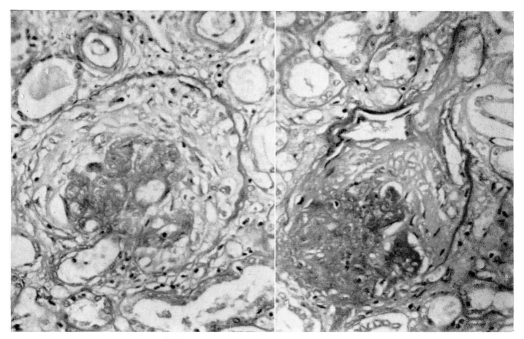

Fig. 4.36. Glomerulonephritis with crescents. Case 13. Autopsy kidney 4 months after first biopsy. Bowman's space obliterated by fibrous tissue. Shrunken glomerular tuft and basement membrane of Bowman's capsule still recognisable. PAS × 250.

Fig. 4.37. Glomerulonephritis with crescents. Case 13. Autopsy kidney 4 months after first biopsy. Fibrous tissue extending from Bowman's space into proximal convoluted tubules. PAS × 250.

deposition of complexes of immunoglobulin and streptococcal antigens. This produces a characteristic appearance demonstrated by immunofluorescence techniques of irregular granular deposits of immunoglobulins and complement (McCluskey, 1971). This pattern is not specific to post-streptococcal disease but is indicative of the deposition of complexes of antigen and antibody in the glomeruli and so is considered to indicate immune complex disease. It is also present in lupus nephritis and malarial glomerulonephritis.

Focal glomerulonephritis

As yet this is a morphological entity but the work of Bates *et al.* (1957) does suggest that at least some of the cases may be caused by a non-streptococcal infective agent.

It seems likely that there are other causes as evidenced by the finding of focal glomerulonephritis in cases of Henoch–Schonlein purpura and polyarteritis nodosa.

Disseminated lupus erythematosus

In groups of cases diagnosed on clinical grounds and on the presence of L.E. cells or antinuclear factor the histological changes are extremely variable and so as a result is the clinical course of renal disease.

Glomerulonephritis with crescents

This morphological group includes cases of different aetiologies. Crescents may be present in a minority of cases of post-streptococcal glomerulonephritis. Crescents may also be present in cases of polyarteritis nodosa but in most cases where crescents are a dominant feature of the

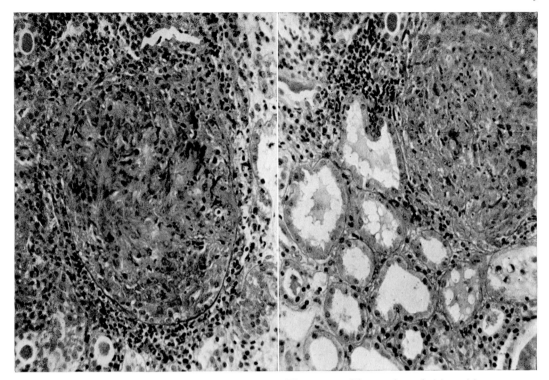

Fig. 4.38. Glomerulonephritis with crescents. Case 14. A large swollen glomerulus. Bowman's space is completely obliterated by a large cellular crescent. PAS × 250.

Fig. 4.39. Glomerulonephritis with crescents. Case 14. The proximal convoluted tubules are dilated and lined by low epithelium probably regenerated. PAS × 250.

disease as in rapidly progressive glomerulonephritis no evidence as to aetiology is present. Nevertheless it is worthwhile separating this group on morphological grounds as the presence of numerous crescents in general indicates a poor prognosis.

Membranous nephropathy

This is a distinct morphological entity with a characteristic long unremitting clinical course. The morphological changes in the glomeruli also follow a characteristic course with time. The consistent presence of immunoglobulins and complement in the glomeruli on immuno-fluorescence probably indicates an immune mechanism but its nature is unknown.

'Minimal change' glomerulonephritis

This is also a distinct morphological entity with a characteristic clinical course and response to treatment and although most cases can be readily diagnosed, in a few instances difficulties arise in distinguishing such cases from mild proliferative glomerulonephritis or from early membranous nephropathy. The distinction from early membranous nephropathy is helped by examining 1 μm sections stained by the PA silver technique and as has been suggested by McCluskey (1971) by immunofluorescence. Membranous nephropathy shows deposits of IgG and complement whereas 'minimal change' glomerulonephritis does not. The recent claim that 'minimal change' glomerulonephritis shows characteristic deposits of IgE (Gerber and Paronetto, 1971) requires confirmation.

Membranoproliferative and lobular glomerulonephritis

These two conditions are morphological variations of the same basic condition consisting of proliferation of predominantly mesangial cells with formation of fibrillar and hyaline interstitial deposits. It has a characteristic very slowly progressive course with typical immunological changes. There has been some published evidence that lobular glomerulonephritis is a late result of post-streptococcal glomerulonephritis but recent studies of membranoproliferative glomerulonephritis have not borne this out.

REFERENCES

ALLEN, A. C. (1962). *The Kidney*, 2nd edition. Churchill, London, p. 258.

BARIÉTY, J., DRUET, PH., SAMARCQ, P. and LAGRUE, G. (1969). *J. Urol. Nephrol.* **75**, 627.

BARIÉTY, J., DRUET, PH., LOIRAT, PH. and LAGRUE, G. (1971). *Path. Biol.* **19**, 259.

BATES, R. C., JENNINGS, R. B. and EARLE, D. P. (1957). *Amer. J. Med.* **23**, 510.

BERGER, J., DE MONTERA, H. and GALLE, P. (1961). *Arch. Anat. path.* **9**, 311.

CAMERON, J. S., GLASGOW, E. F., OGG, C. S. and WHITE, R. H. R. (1970). *Brit. med. J.* **4**, 7.

DODGE, W. F., SPARGO, B. H., BASS, J. H. and TRAVIS, L. B. (1968). *Med. (Balt.)* **47**, 227.

EHRENREICH, T. and CHURG, J. (1968). *Path. Ann.* **3**, 145.

ELLIS, A. (1942). *Lancet* **i**, 1.

GERBER, M. A. and PARONETTO, F. (1971). *Lancet* **i**, 1097.

GOTOFF, S. P., FELLERS, F. X., VAWTER, G. F., JANEWAY, C. A. and ROSEN, F. S. (1965). *New Engl. J. Med.* **273**, 524.

HEPTINSTALL, R. H. and JOEKES, A. M. (1961). *Renal Biopsy*, Ciba Foundation Symposium. Churchill, London, p. 194.

HERDMAN, R. C., PICKERING, R. J., MICHAEL, A. F., VERNIER, R. L., FISH, A. J., GEWURZ, H. and GOOD, R. A. (1970). *Med. (Balt.)* **49**, 207.

JENNINGS, R. B. and EARLE, D. P. (1961). *J. Clin. Invest.* **40**, 1525.

KUSHNER, D. S., ARMSTRONG, S. H., DUBIN, A., SZANTO, P. B., MARKOWITZ, A., MADUROS, B. P., LEVINE, J. M., RIVER, G. L., GYNN, T. N. and PENDRAS, J. P. (1961). *Med. (Balt.)* **40**, 203.

LAWRENCE, J. R., POLLAK, V. E., PIRANI, C. L. and KARK, R. M. (1963). *Med. (Balt.)* **42**, 1.

MCCLUSKEY, R. T. (1971). *J. exp. Med.* **134**, 242S.

MCCLUSKEY, R. T. and BALDWIN, D. S. (1963). *Amer. J. Med.* **35**, 213.

MANDALENAKIS, N., MENDOZA, N., PIRANI, C. L., and POLLAK, V. E. (1971). *Med. (Balt.)* **50**, 319.

MUEHRCKE, R. C., KARK, R. M., PIRANI, C. L. and POLLAK, V. E. (1957). *Med. (Balt.)* **36**, 1.

RAMMELKAMP, C. H., JR. (1953). *Proc. intern. Med. Chic.* **19**, 371.

SALLE, B., MAMELLE, J. C. and LADREYT, J. P. (1968). *Schweiz. med. Wschr.* **98**, 917.

TRESER, G., EHRENREICH, T., ORES, R., SAGEL, I., WASSERMAN, E., and LANGE, K. (1969). *Pediatrics* **43**, 1005.

WEST, C. D., MCADAMS, A. J., MCCONVILLE, JANICE M., DAVIS, N. C. and HOLLAND, N. H. (1965). *J. Pediat.* **67**, 1089.

5

Renal Lesions in Diabetes Mellitus

As the death rate from infective complications in diabetes mellitus falls so deaths due to non-infective complications become proportionately more important. The renal complications are important amongst these.

Tubular lesions

The first structural change described in the kidney in diabetes mellitus was glycogen infiltration of the tubular cells. The changes can readily be recognised in haematoxylin- and eosin-stained sections. The cytoplasm of the affected cells appears clear and completely empty, much clearer than in any other condition (fig. 5.1). In biopsy specimens some glycogen is preserved and stains positively with the PAS stain (fig. 5.2). It is readily removed from the section by pre-treatment with salivary diastase. In sections the tubules affected appear to be in the medulla but the cells are so altered that it is not possible to identify what part of the nephron is involved. Microdissection studies (Ritchie and Waugh, 1957) have shown that the lesions are localised to the terminal straight segments of the proximal convoluted tubules with occasional extensions

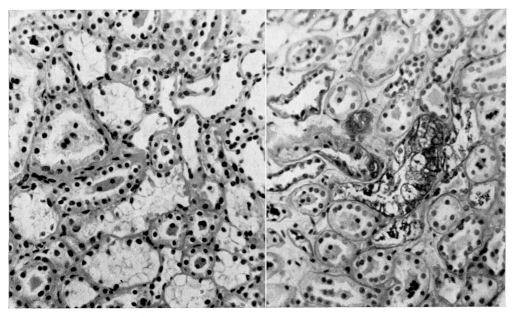

Fig. 5.1. Diabetic nephropathy. Several tubules in the medulla showing glycogen storage. Tubular cells swollen and empty-looking. HE × 250.

Fig. 5.2. Diabetic nephropathy. Glycogen in tubule stained with PAS × 250.

into the adjacent portion of the thin loop of Henle. These studies also showed that the nephrons of the outer part of the cortex with short loops of Henle do not develop this change.

It is said to occur only in uncontrolled diabetes. The biopsy illustrated was taken from a young unstable diabetic who was admitted in ketosis shortly before the biopsy was performed. It appears to be a highly specific lesion being found only in diabetics. As far as is known it produces no functional change. It has been suggested that the lesion results from absorption of large amounts of glucose (Oliver, 1950) but there is little to support this.

Diabetic glomerulosclerosis

The most important renal lesions in diabetes mellitus occur in the glomerulus. Kimmelstiel and Wilson in 1936 described the nodular lesion now known by their names. It is a highly characteristic lesion consisting of a round or oval nodule, acellular and often laminated in appearance. The nodules vary in size from about one-quarter to one-third the diameter of the glomerular tuft. There may be only one in a tuft (fig. 5.3) or up to four or five. The nodules occur virtually only in diabetes mellitus.

The diffuse form of diabetic glomerular disease is much less specific. In fact in the early stages of the disease it is difficult to draw a definite line between normal and abnormal. The process begins at the centres of the glomerular lobules. The cells in this area increase slightly in number and become surrounded by irregular deposits of material that in ordinary sections appear hyaline (fig. 5.4). However, in thin sections stained by the PA silver method it can be seen to consist of a closely woven irregular felt work of fibres (figs. 5.5–5.8, cf. 5.9 showing a normal glomerulus). As the disease progresses the number of cells slowly increases as does the amount of material about them. In addition the peripheral basement membrane becomes thickened and often irregularly crenated. As the amount of material in the lobular centres becomes greater the deposits come to resemble more and more Kimmelstiel–Wilson nodules (fig. 5.10) and it seems probable, as suggested by Allen (1962), that the nodules result from the same process that causes the diffuse change.

These observations, based on simple qualitative examination of renal biopsies have recently been confirmed by quantitative studies. Thus Kimmelstiel and his co-workers (Kawano et al., 1969) measured the mean mesangial area by a planimeter method. They found in normals the mean mesangial area was 6·76 per cent of the total glomerular area. In diffuse diabetic glomerulosclerosis it increased to 17·25 per cent and in nodular lesions it increased to 23·7 per cent. Wehner (1968) and Wehner and Anders (1969) used a different technique, estimating the various areas by point-counting. Their figures for the mean mesangial area as a percentage of the total glomerular area are, in normals 6·2 per cent, in diffuse diabetic glomerulosclerosis 12·7 per cent and in nodular lesions 20·7 per cent. In addition Kawano et al. (1969) found a relative increase in mesangial cells which they suggest may precede the increase in mesangial matrix but in the later stages a greater amount of mesangial matrix is formed so that the number of mesangial nuclei per unit area of mesangial matrix is reduced. There has been considerable discussion re-regarding the relation in time between the onset of diabetes mellitus and the development of the glomerular changes. It has been claimed that glomerular damage is present very early in the disease and may even be present in prediabetes.

Of 37 renal biopsies taken from a series of patients covering a wide age range and having suffered from diabetes mellitus for widely differing times, a number appeared normal when examined by light microscopy. However, when a selected number were examined by electron microscopy (Lannigan et al., 1964) even the earliest cases showed significant thickening of the basement membrane. Similar findings have been reported by Sabour et al. (1962). These findings have given rise to suggestions that as glomerular changes are present so early in the

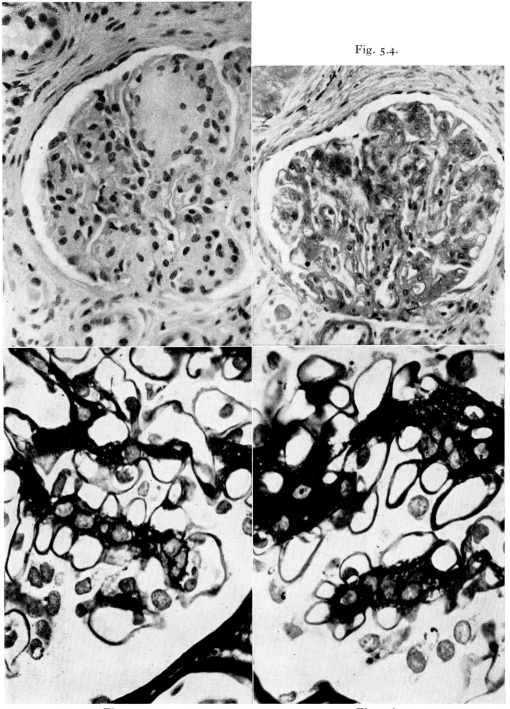

Fig. 5.3.

Fig. 5.4.

Fig. 5.5.

Fig. 5.6.

Fig. 5.3. Diabetic nephropathy. Nodular glomerular lesion. HE × 450.

Fig. 5.4. Diabetic nephropathy. Diffuse glomerular lesion. PAS × 370.

Fig. 5.5. Diabetic nephropathy. Early stage of diffuse glomerular lesion. Increase in cells at centre of lobule surrounded by black staining material. PA silver × 900.

Fig. 5.6. Diabetic nephropathy. Changes seen in fig. 5.5 at more advanced stage. PA silver × 900.

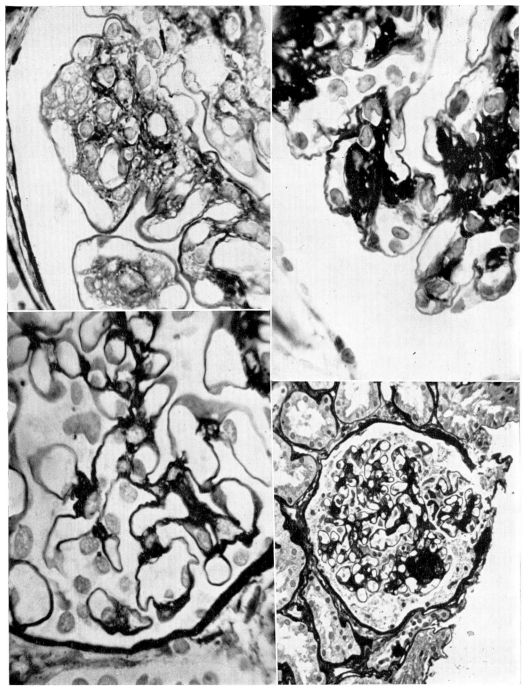

Fig. 5.9.

Fig. 5.10.

Fig. 5.7. Diabetic nephropathy. Greater increase in cells than in figs. 5.5 and 5.6. Material about them can be seen to be fibrillary. PA silver × 900.

Fig. 5.9. Normal glomerulus for comparison with figs. 5.5–5.8. PA silver × 900.

Fig. 5.8. Diabetic nephropathy. Masses of black-staining material at centres of lobules. Peripheral basement membrane crenated. PA silver × 900.

Fig. 5.10. Diabetic nephropathy. Marked thickening at the centres of the lobules. The largest is a nodular lesion. PA silver × 250.

disease they may not be a consequence of the diabetes mellitus but that the diabetes and the glomerular changes may have a single preceding cause. However more recent careful quantitative electron microscope studies (Osterby–Hansen, 1965; Osawa *et al.*, 1966) have shown that the peripheral basement membrane is not thickened in some cases of early juvenile diabetes nor even in some cases of diabetic glomerulosclerosis with nodular lesions.

Clinical correlations

In considering correlations between the development of renal changes and the various aspects of diabetes mellitus it must be borne in mind that electron microscopy will reveal changes in the glomeruli in the very great majority, if not all cases. Studies using light microscopy are therefore considering well established changes.

In general the longer the duration of the diabetes the more advanced are the glomerular changes. The correlation between severity and duration is, however, not very close. There is also wide variation in the rate of development of the lesions. They may progress quite rapidly as the following case illustrates:

Case 1. A boy who developed diabetes in 1953 at the age of 15 was investigated in 1959 when his blood urea was 42 mg/100 ml, his 24-hour urinary protein 1·3–3·9 g and B.P. 160/90. Biopsy at this time (fig. 5.11) showed slight to moderate diffuse changes in the majority of the glomeruli. Rather surprisingly three glomeruli showed small exudative lesions. The diabetes proved rather difficult to control. In 1960 he complained of some deterioration of vision. The 24-hour urinary protein was still about 3·9 g and the B.P. 140/90. In January 1962, in addition to blurring of vision, he complained of swelling of the ankles.

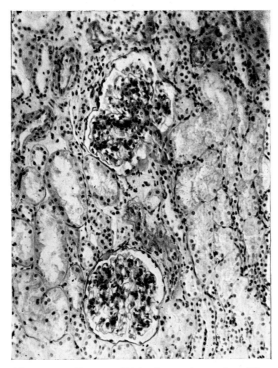

Fig. 5.11. Case 1. Diabetic nephropathy. First biopsy. Two glomeruli showing moderate diffuse change with an atrophic tubule between them. PAS × 150.

The blood urea was 48 mg/100 ml, the creatinine clearance 26 ml/minute and the B.P. 180/110. Biopsy at this time (fig. 5.12) showed definite progression of the glomerular damage during the intervening 32 months. During the ensuing year the hypertension became more severe. Deterioration continued until in October 1963 the creatinine clearance was 10 ml/minute, blood urea 190 mg/100 ml, 24-hour urinary protein 6·4 g and B.P. 230/125. He died in November 1963, 21 months after the second biopsy. The kidneys now showed a very severe diabetic nephropathy (fig. 5.13) with complete hyalinisation of many glomeruli, advanced changes in the remainder with severe tubular atrophy and interstitial fibrosis.

Twenty-eight of the patients on whom renal biopsy had been performed could be divided into two groups, 18 with retinopathy and 10 without. All of those with retinopathy had moderate to severe changes in the kidney. Seven of the 10 without retinopathy had changes but in 4 they were only slight. Eighteen patients had proteinuria (including 5 with no retinopathy) and of these 16 showed glomerular damage. Ten had no proteinuria (including 5 with retinopathy) and 9 of these showed glomerular damage, mild in 4.

The original description of the nodular glomerular lesion drew attention to the associated clinical picture of proteinuria, oedema, and hypertension. However, many cases do not show this and it seems probable that the diffuse lesion is more important functionally than the nodular lesion. This is borne out by the studies of Gellman et al. (1959) who found a close correlation between diffuse diabetic glomerulosclerosis and increasing diastolic blood pressure, proteinuria, blood urea and creatinine, and decreasing serum albumin, urea and creatinine clearances. This was not so with the nodular lesion which they concluded was not functionally important but was important diagnostically.

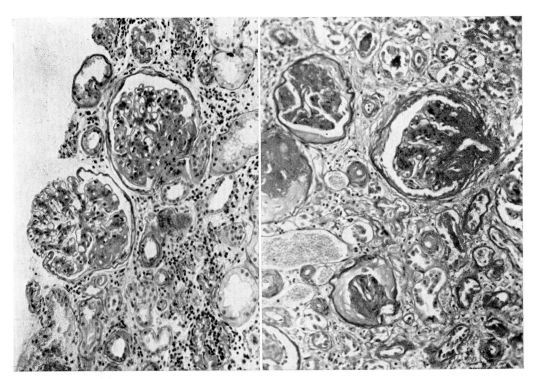

Fig. 5.12. Case 1. Diabetic nephropathy. Second biopsy 32 months after first. Two glomeruli with severe diffuse lesions, atrophy of tubules and interstitial fibrosis. PAS × 150.

Fig. 5.13. Case 1. Diabetic nephropathy. Postmortem kidney 21 months after second biopsy. Very severe glomerular damage. Marked interstitial fibrosis and tubular atrophy. PAS × 150.

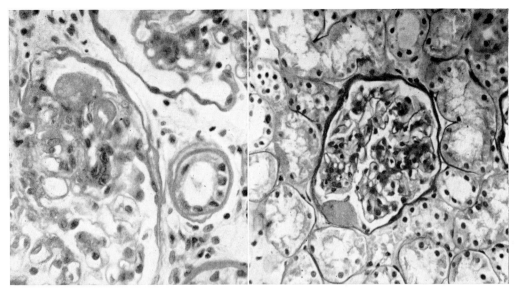

Fig. 5.14. Diabetic nephropathy. Two exudative lesions very close together at the periphery of a glomerulus. PAS × 450.

Fig. 5.15. Diabetic nephropathy. A 'capsular drop' on the inner surface of Bowman's capsule. PAS × 250.

The mode of development

Kimmelstiel and Wilson (1936) described the nodular lesion as intercapillary but Allen (1962) suggested that the change takes place actually in the wall of the capillaries. This difference of opinion is based largely on a misunderstanding of the structure of the glomerular capillaries and particularly of the relation of the mesangium to the capillary lumen. This misunderstanding has now been resolved by electron microscope studies. The mesangium is inside the glomerular

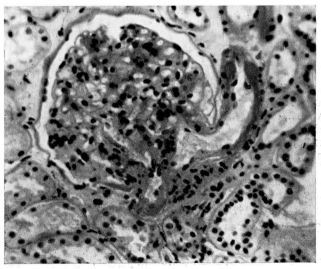

Fig. 5.16. Diabetic nephropathy. A glomerulus with both afferent and efferent arterioles showing hyaline thickening. HE × 250.

capillaries in the sense that it is inside the glomerular basement membrane but it is separated from the capillary lumen by endothelial cells. As Allen (1962) suggested there are changes present in the wall of the capillaries. The glomerular basement membrane is thickened, but the major changes are found in the mesangial areas where there is proliferation of mesangial cells and an increased formation of mesangial matrix much of which resembles nodular crenated basement membrane.

It has been suggested that the glomerular changes result from a deposition of protein or glycoprotein from the plasma. A variety of proteins have been suggested (Le Compte, 1955).

Our light and electron microscope studies (Lannigan *et al.*, 1964), provide strong support for the view that the change is a local one within the glomerulus resulting from proliferation of mesangial cells which then form abnormal amounts of mesangial matrix. The idea is also put forward by Kawano *et al.* (1969).

The exudative lesion and the 'capsular drop'

The exudative lesion consists of a small, brightly eosinophilic mass which is found at the periphery of the glomerular tuft often forming a curved little cap at the outer surface of a capillary loop. It is PAS-positive with a very smooth uniformly stained appearance but often with several vacuoles within it (fig. 5.14). It also very often stains positively for fat and for fibrin. The capsular drop is a small oval deposit on the inner surface of Bowman's capsule (fig. 5.15) which show similar staining reactions.

Although the exudative lesion is common in diabetes mellitus, it occurs in other conditions, particularly the subacute or chronic stage of endothelial cell proliferative glomerulonephritis.

Arteriolar hyalinisation

In diabetic nephropathy of even moderate degree the arterioles always show marked hyaline thickening (fig. 5.16). The changes are most marked in the afferent arteriole, but also affect the efferent arteriole. Efferent arteriolar sclerosis whilst fairly often found in diabetes mellitus occurs only rarely in its absence (Smith, 1955).

The changes are so marked in the later stages of the disease that severe ischaemia must result. It presumably is responsible for the marked tubular atrophy and thickening of the tubular basement membrane that occurs.

REFERENCES

ALLEN, A. C. (1962). *The Kidney*. 2nd. edition. Churchill, London, p. 285.
GELLMAN, D. D., PIRANI, C. L., SOOTHILL, J. F., MUEHRCKE, R. C. and KARK, R. M. (1959). *Med. (Balt.)* **38**, 321.
KAWANO, K., ARAKAWA, M., MCCOY, J., PORCH, J., and KIMMELSTIEL, P. (1969). *Lab. Invest.* **21**, 269.
KIMMELSTIEL, P. and WILSON, C. (1936). *Amer. J. Path.* **12**, 83.
LANNIGAN, R., BLAINEY, J. D. and BREWER, D. B. (1964). *J. Path. Bact.* **88**, 255.
LECOMPTE, P. M. (1955). *J. chron. Dis.* **2**, 178.
OLIVER, J. (1950). *Amer. J. Med.* **9**, 88.
OSAWA, G. KIMMELSTIEL, P. and SEILING, VIRGINIA (1966). *Amer. J. clin. Path.* **45**, 21.
OSTERLEY-HANSEN, RUTH (1965). *Diabetologia* **1**, 97.
RITCHIE, SUSAN and WAUGH, D. (1957). *Amer. J. Path.* **33**, 1035.
SABOUR, M. S., MACDONALD, MARY K. and ROBSON, J. S. (1962). *Diabetes* **11**, 291.
SMITH, J. P. (1955). *J. Path. Bact.* **69**, 147.
WEHNER, H. (1968). *Virchow's Arch. Path. Anat.* **344**, 286.
WEHER, H. and ANDERS, E. (1968). *Ver. dtsch. Ges. Path.* **53**, 380.

6

Pyelonephritis

Acute pyelonephritis

Renal biopsy has not been much used in cases diagnosed clinically as pyelitis. However Hutt and de Wardener (1961) report the interesting finding that in 4 of 10 such cases there were foci of acute inflammation present in the renal cortex, demonstrating that many clinical cases of pyelitis are really cases of pyelonephritis.

I have no experience of renal biopsy in such circumstances but the following case resembling so-called acute diffuse interstitial nephritis is of interest.

Case 1. An 18-year-old West Indian girl developed periorbital oedema and a generalised itching erythematous rash 6 hours after having taken 3 sulphadimidine tablets. She was admitted to hospital where she was found to have a pyrexia of 102–103°F which continued for many days. Her skin rash developed into a generalised exfoliative dermatitis. Her urine output slowly fell until a little more than 3 weeks after admission she became anuric. She was transferred to the General Hospital, Birmingham, for haemodialysis. At this time her blood urea was 420 mg/100 ml. Her right kidney was found to be enlarged. It was explored, a biopsy taken and a ureterostomy performed. Following dialysis her urine flow gradually returned. Sixteen days following the onset of anuria her urinary output was 2 litres in 24 hours, after a further 9 days the blood urea was 51 mg/100 ml and the creatinine clearance 39 ml/minute. Six months after the onset of her illness her blood urea was 44 mg/100 ml and the creatinine clearance 68 ml/minute. Eight years after the biopsy she had normal renal function.

The histological appearances are striking. There is a very heavy cellular interstitial infiltration. The cells present are mainly lymphocytes and histiocytes with small numbers of plasma cells. The glomeruli are normal (fig. 6.1). The tubules are separated by the heavy interstitial inflammatory exudate. The tubular epithelial cells are large with big pale nuclei (fig. 6.2). A number of mitotic figures are present. The appearances suggest regeneration following tubular damage.

Bacteria were isolated from the urine providing some support for the interpretation of the biopsy findings as a bacterial interstitial nephritis. However, the illness began after taking sulphadimidine. The skin disease was clearly a severe hypersensitivity reaction. It would seem very likely that the renal lesion might also be a hypersensitivity reaction. Allen (1962) described such changes occurring in the kidney as a reaction to sulphonamides.

Chronic pyelonephritis

The value of renal biopsy in pyelonephritis is limited because the histological changes seen are irregularly distributed within the kidney and even when changes are found they are difficult to interpret and to distinguish particularly from changes due to hypertension or ischaemia. This difficulty exists even in autopsy material when the whole of both kidneys are available for examination.

Most authors follow more or less closely the criteria laid down by Weiss and Parker (1939). These have recently been reconsidered critically by Kimmelstiel *et al.* (1961). They come to the conclusion that interstitial infiltration with lymphocytes only is of no significance but that an active pleomorphic inflammatory infiltrate, particularly accumulations of polymorphonuclear leukocytes is the safest criterion for the diagnosis of chronic pyelonephritis. In chronic pyelonephritis inflammatory cells particularly polymorphonuclear leukocytes may be absent. They

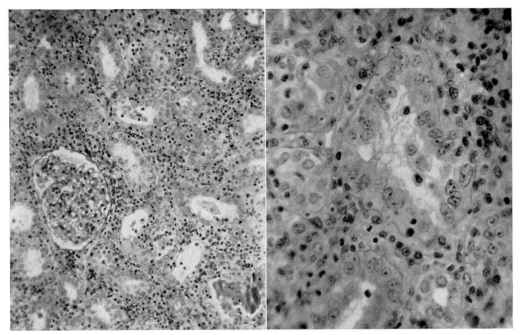

Fig. 6.1. Case 1. ? Interstitial nephritis ? Sulphonamide reaction. There is a heavy interstitial cellular infiltrate, mainly of lymphocytes and histiocytes. The glomerulus is normal. PAS × 150.

Fig. 6.2. Case 1.? Interstitial nephritis? Sulphonamide reaction. The tubular cells are large with pale nuclei. PAS × 450.

then regard the presence of areas of thyroid-like tubular atrophy to be most helpful, provided they are not adjacent to expanding lesions, e.g. cysts and provided the areas are not congenital in origin. Glomerular changes they thought to be of limited value but in general the hyalinised glomeruli in chronic pyelonephritis are irregularly placed and separated by atrophic or dilated tubules. In infarcts the hyalinised glomeruli are closely and solidly packed.

I would agree in general with these ideas. I think the distribution of the changes is probably also helpful. In chronic pyelonephritis the changes tend to be patchy and the patches sharply defined from normal parenchyma. This does not necessarily help in the distinction from an infarct but it does in the more usual problem of the differential diagnosis from the diffuse ischaemic change due to hypertensive vascular disease. In addition in this disorder the sclerosed glomeruli tend to occur in small triangular subcapsular scars so that it is important sometimes to decide where in the cortex the sclerosed glomeruli are. Figure 6.3 is a fairly low power view of a biopsy showing two distinct areas in the kidney. One area shows an almost normal glomerulus with fairly normal tubules about it with moderate interstitial fibrosis. In the other half are 2 glomeruli with marked periglomerular fibrosis, interstitial fibrosis with marked tubular atrophy and heavy lymphocytic infiltration.

This biopsy is from a woman of 53 years (Case 2) who had had over the previous 12 months 4 attacks of right loin pain, haematuria, frequency and dysuria with occasional pyrexia. *B. proteus* was isolated from the urine and also from the renal biopsy. The blood pressure was 145/85, serum creatinine 2·68 mg/100 ml and the creatinine clearance 23 ml/minute.

Figure 6.4 shows a slightly higher power view of the scarred area with crowded completely hyalinised glomeruli. There are small atrophic tubules in the fibrous tissue between the tufts.

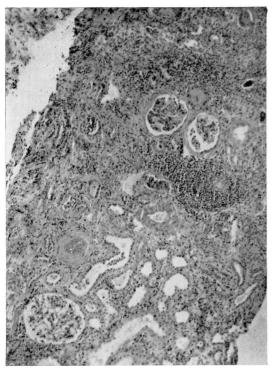

Fig. 6.3. Case 2. Chronic pyelonephritis. Area of severe interstitial fibrosis, complete tubular atrophy, periglomerular fibrosis, and heavy lymphocytic infiltration sharply demarcated from less severely affected area. PAS × 100.

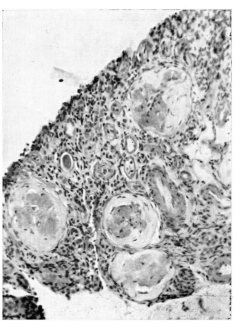

Fig. 6.4. Case 2. Chronic pyelonephritis. Scarred area. Completely hyalinised tufts. Marked interstitial fibrosis in which are very small atrophic tubules. PAS × 150.

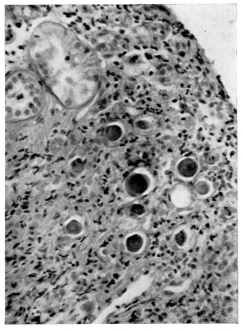

Fig. 6.5. Case 2. Chronic pyelonephritis. Atrophic tubules containing casts. PAS × 250.

Figure 6.5 again from the same biopsy shows thyroid-like atrophy of tubules with atrophic tubules containing casts.

Incidence of positive biopsies in pyelonephritis

The reported incidence of positive findings in clinical cases of pyelonephritis varies widely. This obviously could be affected by factors influencing either the clinical diagnosis or the histological interpretation. A low incidence of positive biopsy findings might result from mistakes in clinical diagnosis including in the series cases that did not have pyelonephritis or from a cautious approach to histological findings accepting only obvious cases. In the reverse way including only very obvious advanced clinical cases of pyelonephritis or accepting questionable histological evidence could increase the incidence of positive biopsy findings.

Leather (1963) performed biopsies in 15 of a series of 30 cases of chronic pyelonephritis diagnosed using clinical and laboratory methods, including the pyrogen or steroid test. In only 4 could a conclusive histological diagnosis be made. In a further 9 the biopsy findings, although not conclusive, supported the diagnosis. In one case normal kidney was found and in the last case the specimen was too small.

Hutt and de Wardener (1961) performed renal biopsies on 60 patients. Twenty-seven were suffering from symptomless proteinuria or hypertension and 6 of these had positive biopsies. Thirty-three had histories suggestive of chronic pyelonephritis and 6 of these also had positive biopsies. Seven of the 33, in addition to a history of pyelonephritis, had abnormal intravenous pyelograms and 3 of these had positive biopsies.

The results of Brun and Raaschou (1961) show a very much higher incidence of positive biopsy findings. They performed biopsies on 78 patients in whom a clinical diagnosis of chronic pyelonephritis had been made and found 'histological changes compatible with the diagnosis of pyelonephritis (acute, recurrent or chronic)' in 73. In 6 of the 78 the diagnosis was originally suggested by histological changes found in the biopsy but even if these are excluded it still makes 67 positive biopsies out of 72. Forty-eight of the patients with renal function below 20 per cent all showed 'pathological renal tissue in the biopsy'.

The conclusion they come to is that nearly all cases of clinical pyelonephritis with impaired renal function show definite histological changes.

The reasons for the differences in results in these series is not certain. As quoted above Brun and Raaschou (1961) include as positive biopsies showing 'histological changes compatible with the diagnosis of pyelonephritis (acute, recurrent or chronic)'. Such an assessment of results might bring Leather's figures up to 13 positive out of 15. The Danish series also included a much larger proportion of cases with impaired renal function, 47 of the 78 had creatinine clearances of less than 20 ml/minute, whereas only one of Hutt and de Wardener's series had a creatinine clearance below 20 ml/minute. Bucht (1961) in the discussion of these papers also claimed that Danish biopsies were as much as ten times bigger than British biopsies!

REFERENCES

ALLEN, A. C. (1962). In *The Kidney*. Churchill, London, p. 404.
BRUN, C. and RAASCHOU, F. (1961). In *Renal Biopsy*. Ciba Foundation Symposium. Churchill, London, p. 245.
BUCHT, H. (1961). In *Renal Biopsy*. Ciba Foundation Symposium. Churchill, London, p. 274.
HUTT. M. S. R. and DE WARDENER, H. A. (1961). In *Renal Biopsy*. Ciba Foundation Symposium. Churchill, London, p. 262.
KIMMELSTIEL, P., KIM. O. J., BERES, J. A. and WELLMANN, K. (1961). *Amer. J. Med.* **30**, 589.
LEATHER, H. M. (1963). *Brit. med. J.* **1**, 440.
WEISS, S. and PARKER, F. (1939). *Med. (Balt.)* **18**, 221.

7

The Kidney and Hypertension

The first systematic study employing renal biopsies is the now classical study of Castleman and Smithwick (1943) into the state of the kidney arterioles in hypertension. They examined renal biopsies taken during splanchnic sympathectomy for hypertension in a series of 100 patients. The object of the investigation was to establish whether the vascular changes found at autopsy in these patients was the cause or the result of their hypertension. They found from their study that hypertension was present before the vascular changes and so concluded they were probably the result of the hypertension. More recently Smithwick with other collaborators has reported a similar study on 1,350 biopsies again taken during sympathectomy for hypertension (Sommers, Pelman and Smithwick, 1958). They interpret the appearances as indicating that vascular spasm is present before structural changes occur. The structural changes when they have developed cause secondary renal changes which may then maintain or accelerate the hypertension. Heptinstall (1954) has made a similar study of renal biopsies taken during sympathectomy. His findings were essentially the same. He found in addition that arteriolar necrosis was confined to those cases with the highest blood pressures. The presence of advanced vascular changes did not necessarily rule out a reduction in blood pressure following the sympathectomy.

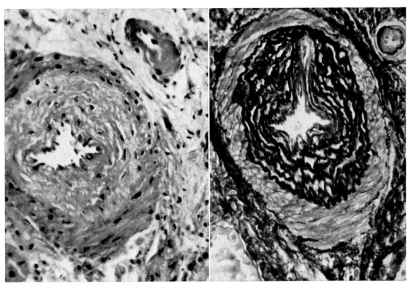

Fig. 7.1 A small muscular artery in a renal biopsy in essential hypertension. There is a marked fibrous intimal thickening. PAS × 235.

Fig. 7.2. The same artery at a different level stained to show the great number of elastic fibres in the intima. Elastic VG × 235.

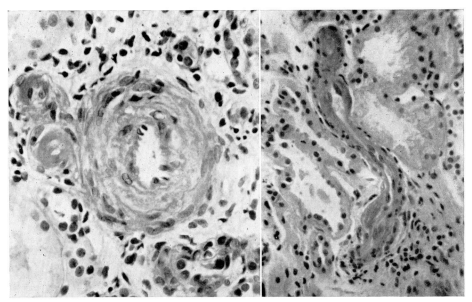

Fig. 7.3. Interlobular artery showing moderate hyperplasia of media and intimal fibrosis. Two adjacent arterioles show hyaline thickening of their walls. PAS × 450.

Fig. 7.4. Longitudinal section of arteriole with hyaline thickened wall. PAS × 250.

One of the important functions of biopsy in cases of hypertension is to exclude any renal cause. This can be done fairly certainly in the case of glomerulonephritis. It may be much more difficult to exclude pyelonephritis.

Whatever the cause of the hypertension provided it has been present for sufficiently long changes will be present in the small muscular arteries of the renal cortex and the arterioles.

In the muscular arteries the media becomes thickened but the most readily recognised change occurs in the intima which becomes markedly thickened. This thickening is due to proliferation of fibrous tissue (fig. 7.1) but also to new formation of elastic tissue internal to the elastic lamina (fig. 7.2). The walls of the arterioles which normally consist of smooth muscle become replaced by acellular hyaline material which is strongly PAS positive (fig. 7.3 and fig. 7.4). This change which affects predominantly the afferent arteriole is found in subjects without hypertension and its incidence increases with age. Its incidence and severity are however increased by hypertension (Smith, 1955).

The effect of these vascular changes is to impair very gradually the blood supply. The impairment is most evident at the periphery of the areas supplied so that multiple little regularly spaced triangular areas of fibrosis develop beneath the capsule. Often tubules cannot be recognised within the fibrous scar but one or two hyalinised glomeruli closely grouped together are usually seen. In these fibrosed glomeruli the shrunken glomerular tuft can be recognised as can the basement membrane of Bowman's capsule. Bowman's space is completely filled by acellular fibrous tissue (fig. 7.5).

Malignant hypertension

In this condition the characteristic lesion, in fact the histological finding by which by definition the diagnosis is made, is necrosis of the arterioles. The prognosis in this condition used to be

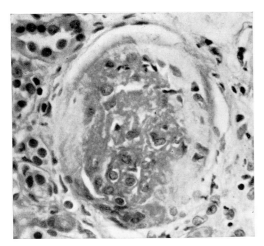

Fig. 7.5. Ischaemic atrophy of a glomerulus. PAS × 450.

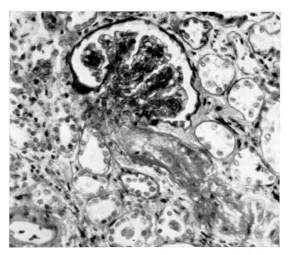

Fig. 7.6. The afferent arteriole appears occluded by thrombus and haemorrhage in its wall. PAS × 250.

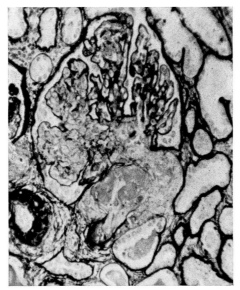

Fig. 7.7. Necrosis of afferent arteriole with thrombosis extending into glomerular tuft. PA silver × 250.

very poor but with modern treatment it is somewhat improved. When such lesions are found in a biopsy they may be difficult to interpret. In one such biopsy in a young woman of 23 I found many thrombi in afferent arterioles extending into glomeruli. Because of this I was initially led into making a diagnosis of thrombotic thrombocytopaenic purpura. However careful examination of the biopsy shows haemorrhagic necrosis of afferent glomerular arterioles (fig. 7.6). This is particularly evident in PA silver preparations where the destruction of the arteriolar is evident. The distension of the glomerular capillaries with resulting rounding of their outlines is also well seen (fig. 7.7.)

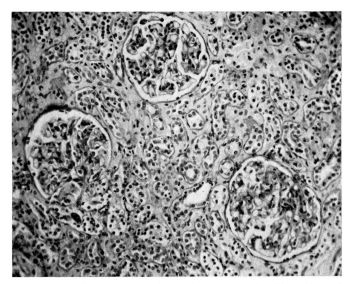

Fig. 7.8. Nephrectomy specimen from case of unilateral renal artery obstruction. Atrophy of tubules, interstitial fibrosis and good preservation of glomeruli. PAS × 150.

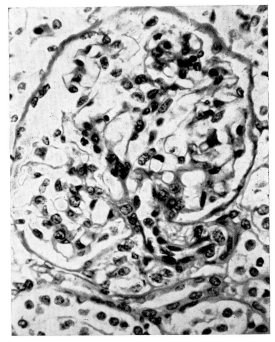

Fig. 7.9. Glomerulus from same specimen as fig. 7.8 showing hyperplasia of juxtaglomerular apparatus. PAS × 450.

This biopsy is from a young woman of 23 who at the age of $18\frac{1}{2}$ was found to have diabetes mellitus. Three years later she developed tuberculous pleural effusions. After another 18 months she developed an illness clinically diagnosed as disseminated lupus erythematosus and L.E. cells were found in the blood. However she developed severe hypertension 210/120 and uraemia and died. At post-mortem no evidence of disseminated lupus erythematosus was found. Histological examination showed widespread necrotising arteriolitis in the renal arterioles.

Unilateral renal artery obstruction and hypertension

Interest in unilateral renal artery obstruction as a cause of hypertension was first stimulated by the work of Goldblatt (1937). Interest has recently intensified as a result of advances in vascular surgery, radiology and clearance techniques for diagnosis. It must be quite a rare cause of hypertension but it is important as the hypertension may be cured by surgical measures, either removing the kidney or restoring its blood supply by vascular surgery.

The effect on the kidney of chronic arterial obstruction is rather variable, but in my experience the commonest effect is a symmetrical reduction in size of the kidney with surprisingly little granularity of the surface. The histological appearances are characteristic. The glomeruli are well preserved. The tubules are atrophic with a diffuse fibrosis about them (fig. 7.8). In some cases there is hyperplasia of the juxtaglomerular apparatus (fig. 7.9). This is thought to be stimulated by the ischaemia to produce renin and so cause the hypertension. Turgeon and Sommers (1961) made a quantitative study of the juxtaglomerular apparatus in a series of these cases and found high juxtaglomerular apparatus cell counts in cases of shorter duration. The patients were younger and had a favourable response to nephrectomy.

REFERENCES

CASTLEMAN, B. and SMITHWICK, R. H. (1943). *J. Amer. med. Ass.* **121**, 1256.
GOLDBLATT, H. (1937). *Ann. intern. Med.* **11**, 69.
HEPTINSTALL, R. H. (1954). *Brit. Heart. J.* **16**, 133.
SMITH, J. P. (1955). *J. Path. Bact.* **69**, 147.
SOMMERS, S. C., PELMAN, A. S. and SMITHWICK, R. H. (1958). *Amer. J. Path.* **34**, 685.
TURGEON, CLAIRE and SOMMERS, S. C. (1961). *Amer. J. Path.* **38**, 227.

8

Miscellaneous Conditions

In this chapter have been gathered together a number of unrelated conditions most of which are somewhat unusual but of considerable interest. It includes several cases of nephrocalcinosis in one of which, due to sarcoidosis there was a proximal tubular defect. A further case of acquired proximal tubular defect due to myelomatosis is then described and finally several different tubular lesions are described.

Nephrocalcinosis

Deposition of calcium in the kidney results from a variety of conditions in which the serum calcium is raised and in which there is generally but not invariably hypercalcuria. It can occur for example in parathyroid adenoma, vitamin D intoxication, multiple osteolytic secondary deposits of carcinoma or prolonged immobilisation. In most cases the deposits of calcium are only found on histological examination but in parathyroid adenoma they may produce serious renal damage which can cause death even after the tumour has been removed. Two examples of nephrocalcinosis are illustrated here, one resulting from chronic alkalosis, the other from sarcoidosis.

The so-called milk-alkali syndrome was first described by Burnett *et al.* (1949). They described 6 patients all with renal failure and all with some evidence of disturbance of their calcium metabolism. There was a raised serum calcium in 5 and evidence of deposition of calcium in the tissues detected as band keratopathy in all 6 cases. All 6 patients had had ulcer symptoms for periods of from 2 to 30 years and all had taken excessive amounts of milk and alkali.

Case 1. A man of 57 had complained of pain after food for 2 years. It had been more severe for the 2 weeks before admission. He was found to have a duodenal ulcer. His blood urea was 242 mg/100 ml and creatinine clearance 9·5 ml per minute. A renal biopsy shows many small deposits of calcium in the medulla where there is also diffuse interstitial fibrosis (fig. 8.1). There are giant cells of foreign body type about many of the deposits (fig. 8.2). The cortex shows a small area of scarring suggestive of chronic pyelonephritis.

Sarcoidosis

It is now well known that the serum calcium may be raised in sarcoidosis and that there may be an increased urinary output of calcium. Such cases are sometimes mistakenly diagnosed as suffering from hyperparathyroidism. Sometimes in such cases calcium may be deposited in the kidney and may eventually cause renal failure. Scholz and Keating (1956) described 8 cases of sarcoidosis with renal complications. In 5 cases calculi were present. The sixth case, the only one in which the kidney was examined histologically, showed nephrocalcinosis. Renal insufficiency was present in 2 cases.

It is difficult to know how commonly this complication occurs in sarcoidosis. Of 52 cases seen at the Massachusetts General Hospital 4 had renal functional impairment, and of these 3 had raised serum calcium levels of from 12 to 16·5 mg/100 ml. Nephrocalcinosis was also present in

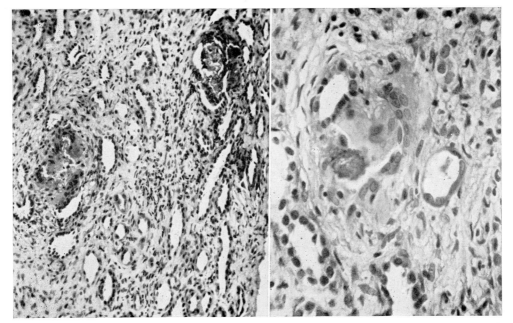

Fig. 8.1. Milk-alkali syndrome. Case 1. Two deposits of calcium in the medulla with diffuse interstitial fibrosis. HE × 150.

Fig. 8.2. Milk-alkali syndrome. Case 1. A small deposit of calcium with foreign body giant cell. HE × 450.

one case of a series of 90 from the Johns Hopkins Hospital. The patient died in uraemia with a serum calcium of 17·4 mg/100 ml (Longcope and Freiman, 1952).

Renal biopsies from 2 cases of sarcoidosis are illustrated here.

Case 2. A woman of 39 was referred to the diabetic clinic because of glycosuria. She had been complaining of loss of weight, thirst, breathlessness and tiredness. She did not have diabetes mellitus. The glycosuria was found to be renal in origin. She also had an aminoaciduria, a hyperchloraemic acidosis with a failure to produce a urine more acid than pH 6. There was also some impairment of urinary concentration. The blood urea was 100–120 mg per 100 ml and the creatinine clearance 10 ml per minute. A liver biopsy shows typical sarcoid follicles. A few months later a renal biopsy was performed. It also shows typical epithelioid and giant cell follicles of sarcoidosis (fig. 8.3). There are quite numerous deposits of calcium mainly in the collecting tubules in the medulla often with what appear to be foreign body giant cells about them (fig. 8.4). There is diffuse interstitial fibrosis in the cortex separating the proximal convoluted tubules. The epithelium of these tubules is abnormal consisting of low cubical cells with no apparent brush border (fig. 8.5).

She was treated with steroids and her renal function improved considerably. Fifteen months after first attending the clinic the blood urea was 60 mg/100 ml and the creatinine clearance had risen to 61 ml/minute. Unfortunately at this time she developed a right sphenoidal ridge meningioma which was successfully operated upon. Eight months later her improvement had been maintained. The blood urea was 49 mg/100 ml.

Five years after the biopsy she still had evidence of renal tubular dysfunction with tubular proteinuria and glycosuria. The blood urea and serum creatinine were normal, B.P. 130/80.

Eight years after the biopsy she was clinically well and her steroid therapy had been stopped for a year.

Case 3. A 34-year-old West Indian bus driver complained of painful joint swellings for about 1 year. He was found to have subcutaneous deposits of calcium about his elbows, shoulders and left thumb. His liver and spleen were enlarged. The serum calcium was 13·7 mg/100 ml, phosphorus 4·2–5·4 mg/100 ml, creatinine 5·1 mg/100 ml. There was a generalised aminoaciduria. In the liver biopsy there are

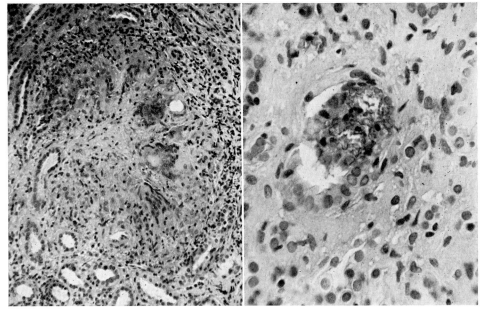

Fig. 8.3. Sarcoidosis. Case 2. A giant cell and epithelioid cell follicle. HE × 150.

Fig. 8.4. Sarcoidosis. Case 2. A deposit of calcium in a collecting tubule. HE × 450.

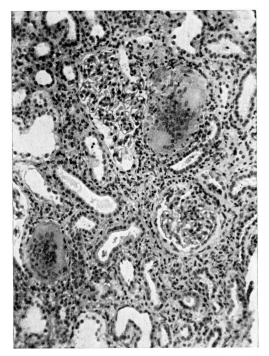

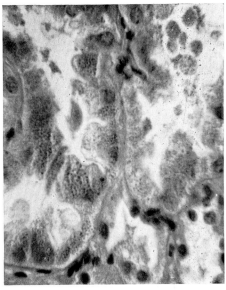

Fig. 8.5. Sarcoidosis. Case 2. Giant cells in renal cortex. Interstitial fibrosis. Proximal tubules lined by rather low simple epithelium. HE × 150.

Fig. 8.6. Sarcoidosis. Case 3. Proximal convoluted tubules showing exceedingly numerous PAS positive droplets. PAS × 450.

typical sarcoid follicles. There are no follicles in the kidney and only one small deposit of calcium. A striking feature, which may have some relevance to the aminoaciduria, is the presence of great numbers of droplets in the epithelial cells of the proximal convoluted tubules. They are smaller and more eosinophilic than the usual hyaline droplets (fig. 8.6).

Nine years after the biopsy his blood urea varied between 55 and 75 mg/100 ml. His serum calcium was within normal limits.

It is interesting that both these cases in addition to renal failure with nitrogen retention had defects of function of their proximal convoluted tubules.

The obvious assumptions have been made that impairment of renal function in sarcoidosis is due either to great numbers of follicular giant cell systems in the renal parenchyma or to deposition of calcium in the kidney. These 2 cases complicate the picture somewhat with the rather unexpected finding of a proximal convoluted tubular defect and in the second case the absence of follicular giant cell systems in the kidney and the presence of only a very small amount of calcium.

Coburn et al. (1967) have reviewed the problem of the renal complications of sarcoidosis and confirm the wide variety of lesions that may be found and the difficulty of fully explaining them.

Multiple myelomatosis

The best known changes found in the kidney in multiple myelomatosis consist of large protein casts mainly in rather dilated distal convoluted tubules with a striking and characteristic giant cell reaction about them. Less often fairly large crystals, slightly larger than the normal lumen are found in the tubular lumen and even more rarely small crystals are found in the cytoplasm of the cells of the proximal convoluted tubules (Sikl, 1949). These changes are a result of the excretion and reabsorption of abnormal protein.

The following case is interesting as the diagnosis for some years was based mainly on the presence of myeloma protein in the urine. No plasma cell tumours or diffuse plasma cell infiltration of the marrow could be demonstrated.

Case 4. A man of 39 complained of tiredness, thirst, low backache, paraesthesia in the hands, occasional morning sickness and frequency for 12 months. He had no anaemia, blood urea 39 mg/100 ml, creatinine clearance 36 ml per minute. He had severe impairment of renal tubular function. There was severe generalised aminoaciduria and glycosuria with normal blood sugar levels. He was excreting 7 g of protein daily in the urine of which about 75 per cent was a gamma-myeloma protein.

The renal biopsy shows a very striking appearance. There is marked interstitial fibrosis (fig. 8.7) and periglomerular fibrosis. The interstitial fibrous tissue shows a moderate lymphocytic infiltration which appears inflammatory in nature. The glomerular tufts apart from the periglomerular fibrosis are normal (fig. 8.7). The proximal convoluted tubules, separated by interstitial fibrosis are lined by large abnormal cells. Their cytoplasm is filled with great numbers of closely packed droplets. The droplets do not stain with eosin or with the PAS stain. They stain lightly with the fuchsin in van Gieson's stain and are Gram positive (figs. 8.8 and 8.9). Amongst the small rounded droplets are a very small number of crystals that show the same staining reactions and are faintly birefringent.

Four years after the biopsy the blood urea was 56 mg/100 ml and the creatinine clearance was 44 ml/min. Radiographs of skull, chest, lumbar spine and pelvis were all normal.

Seven years after the biopsy he developed a swelling at the inner end of the left clavicle and a radiograph showed an osteolytic lesion of the medial third of the left clavicle, collapse of the 5th cervical vertebra and several probable osteolytic lesions in the skull and ribs.

He died 8 years after the biopsy with multiple myelomatosis and renal failure.

The association of multiple myelomatosis with proximal tubular defects of function is rare. Costanza and Smoller (1963) describe a case and refer to 5 other reported cases. In all 3 of the cases in which the kidney was examined there were intracellular crystals in the cells of the proximal convoluted tubules.

7

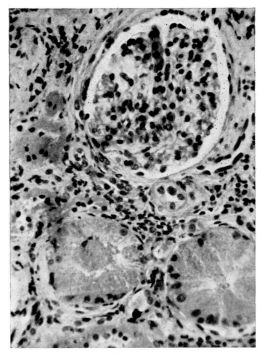

Fig. 8.7. Multiple myelomatosis. Case 4. Marked interstitial fibrosis. Glomerular tuft normal. Tubules lined by large swollen cells. HVG × 250.

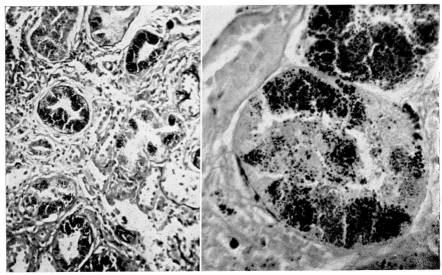

Fig. 8.8. Multiple myelomatosis. Case 4. Tubular cells filled with Gram-positive droplets. Gram's stain × 150.

Fig. 8.9. Multiple myelomatosis. Case 4. Higher power of tubular cells. Gram's stain × 450.

Glomerular embolisation

The glomerular tufts form a prominent part of the capillary bed and have a large blood flow. As might be anticipated small emboli are sometimes held up in the capillaries and are readily seen. In systemic fat embolism fat droplets are commonly found in the glomerular capillaries. Sevitt (1962) advocates renal biopsy as the most reliable means of detecting fat embolism.

Other sorts of emboli may also be readily detected in the glomerular capillaries. Figure 8.10 is a post-mortem kidney showing numerous small clear circular areas. These are silicone emboli. The patient, a child of 8, suffered silicone embolisation from a heart-lung machine whilst being operated on for repair of a ventricular septal defect.

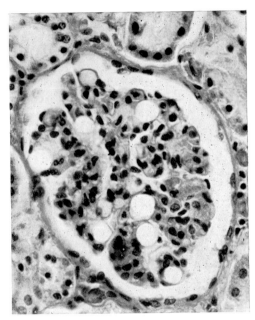 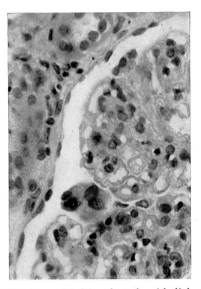

Fig. 8.10. Post-mortem kidney showing many silicone emboli in a single glomerulus. HVG ×?450.

Fig. 8.11. Multinucleated epithelial giant cell in glomerulus in proliferative glomerulonephritis. PAS × 450.

Glomerular epithelial giant cells

Often in proliferative glomerulonephritis the glomerular epithelial cells are enlarged with rather basiphilic cytoplasm. Rarely they become multinucleate (fig. 8.11).

I do not attach any special significance to this change, but regard it as an unusual manifestation of proliferative glomerulonephritis. Montaldo and Ferreli (1963) found similar cells in the glomerulus in a patient who also had tuberculosis and thought that the cells were in some way related to the tuberculosis. I have seen these cells in many cases in which there has been no evidence of tuberculosis.

Tubular regeneration

The proximal convoluted tubules are peculiarly susceptible to a variety of substances that produce in them a specific and severe necrosis, for example, mercury and uranium salts. They react to this necrosis by a very active cellular proliferation. Many mitotic figures are seen in animals recovering from such experimental lesions. It is in fact clear that the total mass of tissue

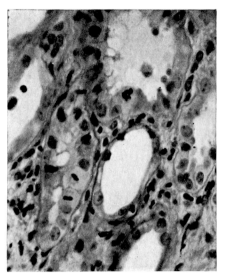

Fig. 8.12. Regenerating tubules showing two mitotic figures. PAS × 450.

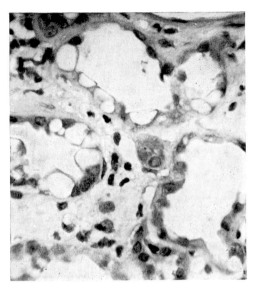

Fig. 8.13. Vacuolar tubular nephropathy due to potassium deficiency. HE × 450.

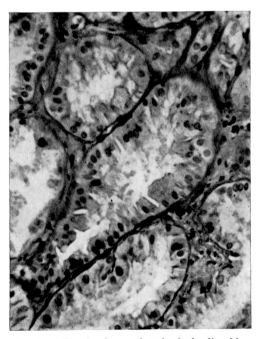

Fig. 8.14. Proximal convoluted tubules lined by clear columnar cells. PAS × 250.

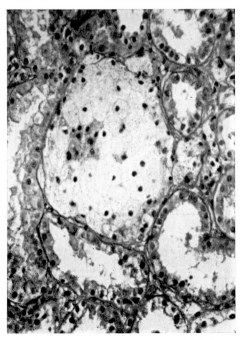

Fig. 8.15. A collection of interstitial foam cells. HE × 250.

made up by the proximal convoluted tubules is very precisely dependent on the metabolic needs of the rest of the body and responds quite rapidly to these needs. Thus Addis (1948) showed that merely by adjusting the amount of protein in the diet one could in rats of the same body weight produce kidneys that varied from 956 mg on a protein free diet to 1,666 mg on a high protein diet. He also showed that following surgical removal of renal tissue the remainder increased in weight very rapidly. Thus after removal of 75 per cent of the kidney tissue the remaining 25 per cent doubled the amount of protein it contained in 5 days. In this rapidly growing kidney remnant there was a disproportionate increase in the size of the proximal convoluted tubules.

In the human the proximal convoluted tubules are equally responsive to damage. Figure 8.12 shows two mitotic figures in tubules regenerating after damage in a case of very severe proliferative glomerulonephritis.

The tubular lesion of potassium depletion

Potassium depletion produces a very characteristic change in the tubular epithelial cells. It consists of the formation of large vacuoles in the cytoplasm. Commonly a single large vacuole is present enlarging and distorting the cell cytoplasm (fig. 8.13). Although the evidence that this change in the human is produced by potassium depletion is good, it has not proved possible to produce it consistently in experimental animals. In fact changes in the collecting tubules consisting of swelling of the cells and cytoplasmic granulation have been more characteristic of experimental potassium depletion.

Columnar epithelium in proximal convoluted tubules

In a few biopsies the proximal convoluted tubules are lined by fairly tall, rather pale, columnar cells (fig. 8.14). The cases I have seen have been so few that it is not possible to discover any reason for this change.

Foam cells

Sharply demarcated round or oval collections of foam cells are commonly found in renal biopsies from cases of nephrotic syndrome (fig. 8.15). It has been suggested that such foci are of significance in the diagnosis of familial glomerulonephritis (Alport's syndrome) but they are so commonly found that I do not think this can be so. Sanerkin (1963) has recently suggested that these collections of foam cells are not interstitial but are confined within the basement membrane of defunct tubules. Some foci of foam cells do appear to be encircled by a ring of fibre but in many deposits this is not so.

REFERENCES

ADDIS, T. (1948). In *Glomerular Nephritis*, Macmillan, New York, p. 58.
BURNETT, C. H., COMMONS, R. R., ALBRIGHT, F. and HOWARD, J. E. (1949). *New Engl. J. Med.* **240**, 787.
COBURN, J. W., HOBBS, C., JOHNSTON, G. S., RICHERT, J. L., SHINABERGER, J. H. and ROSEN, S. (1967). *Amer. J. Med.* **42**, 273.
COSTANZA, D. J. and SMOLLER, M. (1963). *Amer. J. Med.* **34**, 125.
LONGCOPE, W. T. and FREIMAN, D. G. (1952). *Med. (Balt.)* **31**, 1.
MONTALDO, G. and FERRELI, A. (1963). *Virchows Arch. Path. Anat.* **336**, 308.
SANERKIN, N. G. (1963). *J. Path. Bact.* **86**, 135.
SCHOLZ, D. A. and KEATING, F. R. JR. (1956). *Amer. J. Med.* **21**, 75.
SEVITT, S. (1962). In *Fat Embolism*. Butterworths, London, p. 198.
SIKL, H. (1949). *J. Path. Bact.* **61**, 149.

Technical Appendix

(Written in collaboration with Allan Ayres, Chief Technician, and Barrie Sims, Technician, General Hospital, Birmingham)

The aim in preparing sections of renal biopsies is to make the task of diagnosis and assessment of the degree of change as easy as possible. Our present method of investigation includes a plastic embedding technique by which sections of 1 μm thickness can readily be produced but it is appreciated that paraffin wax embedding is still an important and useful method. For this reason the Technical Appendix is divided into two parts. Part I dealing with our own modifications for plastic embedding and staining and Part II with the paraffin wax technique.

There are many points of technique at all steps in processing that are important, but in general the end result should be slides bearing a short run of 6–8 serial sections cut really thin and well stained. It is helpful sometimes in determining the nature of small glomerular lesions to be able to follow them through several serial sections. Many of the judgments made are based on comparisons with previous biopsies, therefore consistency is all important. This must be borne in mind when deciding to adopt the plastic embedding method. Sections cut at 1 μm produce appearances of striking clarity (fig. A.1) even when compared with 4 μm plastic embedded sections (fig. A.2) but the glomeruli appear much less cellular.

PART I   PLASTIC EMBEDDING

Preparation of thin sections using glycol methacrylate (modified from Craig Ruddell, 1967).

Reagents

Mixture A (Infiltrating media)

2-Hydroxyethyl methacrylate	= 80 ml
2-Butoxyethanol	= 8 ml
Benzoyl peroxide	= 0·5 g

Mixture B (Promoter)

NN-Dimethylaniline	= 1 part
Polyethylene glycol '400'	= 8 parts

Fixation The method is compatible with most fixatives.

METHOD

1. Dehydrate to abs. alcohol.
2. Infiltrate with mixture A (2–3 changes).
3. Transfer tissue to aluminium foil tins in a cold-water bath and pour on final plastic soln. Comprising of 42 parts mixture A to 1 part mixture B. Allow to polymerise.
4. Remove foil tins and trim blocks with fine-toothed saw.
5. Attach plastic block to wooden block with ester wax.

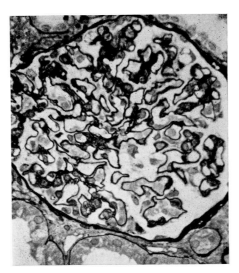

Fig. A.1. 1 μm plastic-embedded section.
P.A. silver × 500 (approx.).

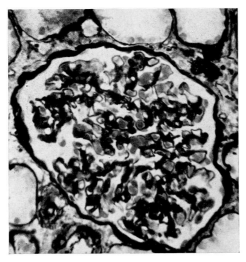

Fig. A.2. 4 μm plastic-embedded section.
Compare with fig. A.1. P.A. silver × 500
(approx.).

6. Gently 'rough cut' to expose tissue.

7. Cut sections with an even steady movement, gently breathing on block to facilitate easier handling of sections.

8. Carefully float on cold water.

9. Pick up sections on clean slides and heat gently over a Bunsen flame until dry.

10. Sections are now ready for staining.

All steps are performed at room temperature.

Notes on Technique

1. The plastic described is harder than the original—giving in our hands more consistent results.

2. Batches of benzoyl peroxide may vary according to supplier. The granular form (Hopkin & Williams, Essex, England) has been found to be most satisfactory.

3. The infiltrating solution should be stored at 4°C, but allowed to warm up to room temperature before use.

4. Mixture B—the promoter—should be prepared just before use. (Care should be taken in handling of all the above solutions as they may cause skin irritation.)

5. Ruddell has used the method successfully after fixation in Zenker's, Carnoy's, formalin, neutral phosphate-buffered formalin, and formalin and glutaraldehyde mixtures with and without CrO_3 or OsO_4.

6. Tissues should not exceed 0·2 cm in thickness for routine work. The largest blocks so far handled have not exceeded $3 \times 2 \times 0·2$ cm.

7. Renal biopsies can be processed within 24 hours.

8. Infiltration is complete when tissue appears partially transparent when held against light.

9. During polymerisation vapour is evolved and the tissue becomes completely transparent. Polymerisation times may vary.

10. For single sections blocks should be trimmed with a leading, pointed 'tongue' of plastic to facilitate easier handling and cutting. For serial work the conventional rectangle is used with a 'sticky wax' trailing the block.

STAINING

Most of the 'routine' methods can be used, e.g., celestin blue, Mayers haemalum & eosin, celestin blue-Mayers haemalum & Van Gieson, PAS, PA silver (Jones, 1957)—but it must be borne in mind that the staining time may have to be prolonged. Alkaline solutions (as in the PA silver method) and prolonged washings (over 12 to 24 hours) tend to detach sections from the slides. Sections can be prevented from becoming detached by coating the 'free' plastic border around the section with shellac varnish. (This does not prevent the section from becoming raised from the slide.) The section, however, can be completely re-attached to the slide by gentle heating (as in Step 9 of the method). For silver methods this is preferably carried out after toning and before fixation.

We have found that the best results with celestin blue Mayers haemalum—Van Gieson and PAS have been attained on 4 μm-thick sections.

The most consistent results with the PAS silver technique have been achieved by using freshly prepared reagents. While giving consistent results in our hands it is appreciated that some difficulty may be encountered in the early stages of working with this method.

PART II   PARAFFIN WAX EMBEDDING

Fixation: Several fixatives are satisfactory.

10% Formal saline (used in this laboratory).

Helly's Fluid. Fixatives containing mercury make it difficult to obtain satisfactory results with the PA silver method.

'Susa'—This fixative appears to produce brighter PAS staining—but it is often more difficult to assess thickening of the glomerular basement membrane than with other fixatives.

Dehydration: Through graded alcohols to abs. alcohol.

Clearing: Equal parts alcohol–chloroform mixture followed by two changes of pure chloroform.

Embedding: Paraffin wax m.p. 56°C–58°C. Two changes. (We have found that 'Paraplast' (Sherwood Medical Industries Inc., St. Louis, U.S.A.) is a most suitable wax.)

This schedule may be carried out on an automatic tissue processor.

Cutting: Sections should be thin. For routine staining methods 4 μm thick. For sections to be stained by the PA silver method sections of 1–2 μm thickness are desirable.

REFERENCES

JONES, D. B. (1957). *Amer. J. Path.* **33,** 313.
RUDDELL, C. (1967). *Stain Technol.* **42,** 119.
RULDELL, C. (1967). *Stain Technol.* **42,** 253.

Index

(Bold numerals indicate illustrations in text)